ESSENTIAL PLAY THERAPY TECHNIQUES

Also Available

Contemporary Play Therapy:
Theory, Research, and Practice
Edited by Charles E. Schaefer and Heidi Gerard Kaduson

Separation Anxiety in Children and Adolescents:
An Individualized Approach to Assessment and Treatment
Andrew R. Eisen and Charles E. Schaefer

Short-Term Play Therapy for Children, Third Edition
Edited by Heidi Gerard Kaduson and Charles E. Schaefer

ESSENTIAL PLAY THERAPY TECHNIQUES

Time-Tested Approaches

Charles E. Schaefer
Donna Cangelosi

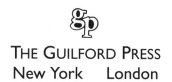

THE GUILFORD PRESS
New York   London

Printed in the United States of America

This book is printed on acid-free paper.

Last digit is print number: 9 8 7 6 5 4

The authors have checked with sources believed to be reliable in their efforts to provide
information that is complete and generally in accord with the standards of practice that are
accepted at the time of publication. However, in view of the possibility of human error or
changes in behavioral, mental health, or medical sciences, neither the authors, nor the editors
and publisher, nor any other party who has been involved in the preparation or publication
of this work warrants that the information contained herein is in every respect accurate or
complete, and they are not responsible for any errors or omissions or the results obtained from
the use of such information. Readers are encouraged to confirm the information contained in
this book with other sources.

Library of Congress Cataloging-in-Publication Data

Schaefer, Charles E.
  Essential play therapy techniques : time-tested approaches / Charles E. Schaefer, Donna Cangelosi.
    pages cm
  Includes bibliographical references and index.
  ISBN 978-1-4625-2449-5 (paperback : acid-free paper)
  1. Play therapy—Methodology.   2. Child psychotherapy.   I. Cangelosi, Donna M.   II. Title.
  RJ505.P6S278 2016
  618.92′891653—dc23
                                                                                    2015029475

To the creators of these
classic play therapy techniques

About the Authors

Charles E. Schaefer, PhD, RPT-S, is Professor Emeritus of Psychology at Fairleigh Dickinson University. He is cofounder and director emeritus of the Association for Play Therapy, which recognized him with its Lifetime Achievement Award. Dr. Schaefer's more than 60 books include *The Therapeutic Powers of Play, Foundations of Play Therapy, Play Therapy with Adolescents,* and *Short-Term Play Therapy for Children, Third Edition.* He maintains a private practice in child psychotherapy in Hackensack, New Jersey.

Donna Cangelosi, PsyD, RPT-S, maintains a private practice with children, adolescents, and adults in Wayne, New Jersey, where she practices psychotherapy, clinical supervision, and parent education. She is coeditor of *Play Therapy Techniques* and *The Playing Cure* and author of *Saying Goodbye in Child Psychotherapy.* Dr. Cangelosi has authored a number of professional articles and chapters on the theory and application of psychodynamic play therapy.

Preface

In essence, play therapy is the use of the therapeutic powers of play to promote healing and growth in clients through a professional relationship. The field of play therapy has benefited from a very wide range of creative play therapy techniques for children. Only a few, however, have stood the test of time and remained popular for an extended period of time. In this book, we consider the select group of classic, time-honored techniques that have remained popular in their original form or in recent variations for at least three decades. In a number of cases, the techniques in this book have been popular for centuries and even millennia. Thus, they can be classified among the "all-time best" play therapy techniques. Fueled by basic human needs, strengths, and interests, they have remained effective across the ages and across cultures. They clearly belong in every play therapist's therapeutic toolbox.

A *technique* can be defined as a concrete procedure applied by a therapist to implement one or more therapeutic change agents. Techniques differ from the strategies that therapists use *in response* to a specific behavior of a client (e.g., limit setting, reflection of feelings, reframing, interpretations). Techniques refer to *therapist-initiated behaviors* that translate abstract theories and change agents into specific, practical interventions. A description of 58 of these basic techniques follows. They were selected not only because of their longevity and popularity, but because of their "user-friendly" simplicity and cost, as well as wide applicability to a range of childhood problems.

We used a transtheoretical approach to obtain the most inclusive list of practical techniques. Thus, we drew from a wide variety of theoretical orientations, including psychoanalytic, Jungian, Adlerian, humanistic, cognitive-behavioral, narrative, Gestalt, solution focused, and prescriptive. Like many therapists, we eclectically selected techniques from diverse theories without espousing or trying to integrate the theories in their entirety (Lazarus, 1981). The basic premise is that the more tools you have available, the more you will be able to meet the varied and individual needs of your clients. Clearly, one method doesn't work for all children or all presenting problems. It is vital for play therapists to have a repertoire of techniques to best meet the needs of all children.

Each technique in the book contains an *Introduction* that provides a historical perspective on the technique, a *Rationale* explaining its therapeutic power(s), a *Description* of how to implement it in play therapy, a review of underlying *Empirical Findings*, and an overview of its *Applications* to specific childhood difficulties and disorders. In addition, recent variations of the core techniques that apply the same basic principles of change are included. As a result, clinicians are provided with hundreds of techniques that can be put right to use in their practice. The techniques are grouped together into the following broad categories: Toy and Object Play, Metaphors and Storytelling, Role Play, Creative Arts, Imagery and Fantasy, Game Play, and Other Techniques.

The techniques contained in this book offer child clinicians a range of time-tested tools to match to the individual needs, interests, and strengths of children. However, no technique will be more important in successful therapy than the quality of the relationship the therapist develops with the child and parent. The better the therapeutic relationship, the greater the therapeutic change one can expect in the child (Kazdin, Whitley, & Marciano, 2006).

This sourcebook of timeless play therapy techniques and their variations should be of interest to beginning and experienced child mental health practitioners from a broad spectrum of theoretical orientations and disciplines, including clinical, counseling, and school psychology; social work; marriage and family therapy; psychiatry; nursing; and child life.

Acknowledgment

We are grateful to our editor at The Guilford Press, Rochelle Serwator, for her support, guidance, and encouragement during all phases of the publishing process.

References

Kazdin, A. E., Whitley, M., & Marciano, P. (2006). Child–therapist and parent–therapist alliance and therapeutic relationship in the treatment of children referred for oppositional, aggressive, and antisocial behavior. *Journal of Child Psychology and Psychiatry, 47*(5), 436–445.

Lazarus, A. (1981). *The practice of multimodal therapy.* New York: McGraw-Hill.

Contents

PART II. METAPHORS AND STORYTELLING TECHNIQUES

PART III. ROLE-PLAY TECHNIQUES

PART IV. CREATIVE ARTS TECHNIQUES

Part One

TOY AND OBJECT PLAY TECHNIQUES

1

Ball Play

BALL TOSS PLAY

Introduction

Ball toss play is one of the earliest and most enduring forms of human play. Prehistoric man played throwing games with sticks, bones, and stones (Reid, 1993). Such activities, which improved the speed and accuracy of throwing an object, were beneficial to survival by primitive people who hunted their food. As early as 2050 B.C.E. playing ball was depicted on Egyptian hieroglyphics. All kinds of balls have been created for this activity, including baseballs, footballs, koosh balls, and beach balls. Since the physical act of throwing and catching a ball gives one kinesthetic, tactile, and visual pleasure, we are hardwired to enjoy it. The goal of playing catch is to have fun while cooperatively keeping a ball going back and forth between two or more participants. In his book *The Ball: Discovering the Object of the Game*, Fox (2012) explains why throwing, catching, bouncing, and hitting a ball has, from our earliest days, been such an integral part of the fun that makes us human. He notes that there are few activities that feel as enjoyable and as deeply satisfying as a good game of catch.

Rationale

The therapeutic benefits of playing catch are numerous. Since it takes into account the child's natural need for activity and movement, it quickly elevates one's mood and strengthens a sense of competence. It can relieve pent-up frustrations and internalized stress. An inherently social activity, it is a way to connect with others through a reciprocal, cooperative action. Early in therapy, ball playing with a child can be used to establish a relaxed, enjoyable atmosphere to develop rapport with a child and facilitate the child's expression of feelings. Ball playing engages the "whole child," including the child's emotions, attention, interests, and strengths.

Description

Ages

Four years and up.

Materials

A number of colorful, soft balls (e.g., foam, Nerf, Koosh, or beach balls). Avoid all balls that could cause pain or damage if thrown hard.

Techniques

Ice-Breaker

Soft ball play can be an effective way to promote positive social interactions among participants in group play therapy. The group therapist begins the activity by stating, "Raise your hand if you would like to play a game of catch. OK, in this game when you catch this ball you say something you like before throwing the ball on to someone else with his/her hand up. Here we go: 'I like chocolates, how about you?'" (The therapist throws the ball to a group member.)

Cooperative Ball Play

As an ice-breaker in a small play therapy group, the therapist tells the group members to try to keep two or more balls (or balloons) in motion together and see how long they can keep the two balls in the air without touching the ground. The therapist times the interaction with a stopwatch. An alternate activity is to give the group a number of "sock balls" to throw into a wastepaper basket. You can make it more challenging by putting the basket on a chair or moving it around the room.

Catch That Feeling

In group therapy, the children are asked to throw a ball back and forth to each other. Each time a ball is caught, the child is directed to express a feeling about an agreed-upon topic, such as what makes him/her happy. For example:

> X: I'm happy we're moving because I like our new house. (*Throws the ball.*)
> Y: You're happy because you like your new house. I'm happy because. . . .

The physical act of throwing a ball back and forth keeps the children focused and the playful atmosphere eases inhibitions about expressing feelings.

Question Ball

This technique involves the use of a beach ball with questions marked on each panel for the "catchee" to answer, such as "Say a nice thing about the person who threw you the ball."

Empirical Findings

Salmon, Ball, Hume, Booth, and Crawford (2008) found that vigorous physical activity, such as ball play, prevented excess weight gain in 10-year-old children.

Applications

Since ball playing is such a familiar and enjoyable activity for children it can be widely used to establish rapport in individual therapy and promote cohesion in child group therapy.

STRESS BALLS

Introduction

A stress ball is a soft ball that fits in the palm of your hand. It is usually 1–3 inches in diameter and made of foam or soft gel. A stress ball could also be made of play dough or modeling clay. The earliest stress balls were Chinese stress balls, which date back to the Sung Dynasty (960–1279 C.E.). Adults would rotate a pair of balls in their hand to help relieve stress and improve hand coordination. Today, Chinese stress balls are made of materials ranging from steel to jade.

Rationale

Therapeutic benefits of stress balls include:

• *Release of physical tension.* Whenever you make a fist, regardless of whether you have something in your hand, you create muscle tension. When you release your grip, your muscles relax. This process can help relax chronically tense muscles and relieve feelings of stress. Thus, providing a child with a stress ball to play with during your intake interview can help relieve the child's tension and anxiety.

• *Mood enhancement.* Squeezing soft stress balls results in pleasurable tactile, kinesthetic, and visual sensations that can boost one's mood.

• *Increased focus.* A hand fidget object such as a stress ball can help children to be less distracted and more focused on classroom instruction. Fidgety children are able to release excess energy in a positive, relaxing way. Children can squeeze the balls under their desks or in their pockets. This activity can help children with attention-deficit disorder (ADD), attention-deficit/hyperactivity disorder (ADHD), and children who are bored or restless focus better.

Description

Ages

Two years and up.

Techniques

Counter to Specific Stressors

Children facing stressful situations, such as a painful medical or dental procedure, can be given a stress ball to help distract and comfort them. Children becoming agitated and upset can also be given a stress ball to calm themselves.

Progressive Muscle Relaxation—for Tweens, Teens, and Adults

Instruction: While slowly and rhythmically squeezing and releasing the stress ball, focus on the physical sensation of muscle tension and relaxation. After a 3-minute workout, switch to your other hand and repeat the exercise. Then tense and relax the other muscle groups in your body, including your facial, shoulder, stomach, thigh, and feet muscles.

Mr. Ugly (Schmidt, 1997)

This technique involves the use of a rubber squeeze toy (i.e., the "Martian Popping Thing") whose eyes, ears, and nose pop out when he is squeezed hard. This is a concrete metaphor for how one's brain feels when it is stressed and overwhelmed. The release of muscle tension from playing with this toy helps reduce one's stress level. The silliness of Mr. Ugly's expression when squeezed enhances the effect.

The child is given the toy and told to squeeze hard, release, and squeeze again a number of times. While the child squeezes the toy, the therapist explains that ugly thoughts or feelings that are located in the child's mind will be squeezed out of the mind and down the neck, across the shoulders, and into the belly of Mr. Ugly. After squeezing to a count of 10, the child is instructed to stop, relax, and take a deep breath. The Mr. Ugly popping toy is useful in group and individual therapy for latency-age children who are under various forms of stress.

Laughing Stress Ball

This stress ball features an added dimension: hysterical laughter when squeezed! It is available from *www.officeplayground.com.*

Empirical Findings

1. Kimport and Robbins (2012) found that squeezing a stress ball for 5 minutes reduced the negative mood of college students. When they were given the instruction to "Hold and squeeze the ball in one hand and then toss it to the other hand, and then repeat this play" for the 5 minutes, the reduction in their negative mood was greater than if they were given no instruction on how to use the stress ball (free play).

2. Studies in the *Journal of Psychosocial Nursing* (2006) reported that using therapeutic touch exercises such as stress balls helped decrease adult anxiety and tension, and assisted in the healing process of wounds.

3. A study by Waller, Kent, and Johnson (2007) found that when a teacher prompted a 14-year-old boy with a fingernail-biting habit to use a stress ball as a replacement for fingernail biting his biting habit decreased significantly.

4. An investigation by Stalvey and Brasell (2006) found that when sixth-grade students were allowed to use stress balls during direct instruction and independent practice the frequency of their distraction incidents decreased. Kinesthetic learners used the stress balls more consistently and their attention spans increased more compared with other learners. However, all types of learners reported that their attitude, attention, writing abilities, and peer interactions improved due to stress ball use.

Applications

Stress balls are commonly used to relieve physical tension and psychological stress in children and adolescents presenting with symptoms of anxiety, obsessive–compulsive disorder (OCD), and trichotillomania; to reduce fidgetiness and distractibility in children with ADD and ADHD; and to lighten children's negative mood.

References

Fox, J. (2012). *The ball: The object of the game.* New York: HarperPerennial.

Hudak, D. (2000). The therapeutic use of ball play in psychotherapy with children. *International Journal of Play Therapy*, 9(1), 1–10.

Kimport, E., & Robbins, S. (2012). Efficacy of creative clay work for reducing negative mood:

A randomized controlled trial. *Art Therapy: Journal of the American Art Therapy Association*, 2(2), 74–79.

Salmon, J., Ball, K., Hume, C., Booth, M., & Crawford, D. (2008). Outcomes of a group-randomized trial to prevent excess weight gain, reduce screen behaviors and promote physical activity in 10-year-old children. *International Journal of Obesity, 32*, 601–612.

Schmidt, M. (1997). Mr Ugly. In H. G. Kaduson & C. E. Schaefer (Eds.), *101 favorite play therapy techniques* (pp. 313–315). Northvale, NJ: Jason Aronson.

Stalvey, S., & Brasell, H. (2006). Using stress balls to focus the attention of sixth-grade learners. *Journal of At-Risk Issues, 12*(2), 7–16.

Waller, R., Kent, S., & Johnson, M. (2007). Using teacher prompts and habit reversal to reduce fingernail biting in a student with attention deficit hyperactivity disorder and a mild intellectual disability. *TEACHING Exceptional Children Plus, 3*(6), 1–8.

2

Plush Doll Play

Introduction

Studies have shown that up to 70% of young children in the Western World develop strong attachments to soft objects such as plush, cuddly toys. These objects, also known as security objects and transitional objects (Winnicott, 1953) are characterized by their soft texture that is reminiscent of being held, comforted, fed, and played with by their mother or caretaker during infancy. During normal development, an infant is likely to become attached to a soft object sometime between the ages of 4 and 12 months. The soft objects seem to provide an added source of comfort for them in falling asleep on their own (Ahluvalia & Schaefer, 1994).

Hong (1978) distinguished between primary and secondary transitional objects. Primary transitional objects are soft, malleable, cuddly attachment objects, such as blankets and pillows, whose onset is usually in the second half of the first year of life and whose use relates to issues of attachment and separation. Bowlby (1969) observed that in the absence of the natural object of attachment, the child may direct behavior to inanimate substitute objects, "instead of to the mother's body, hair, or clothing, clinging may be directed to a blanket or cuddly toy" (p. 312).

Secondary transitional objects refer to soft, cuddly toys, such as teddy bears, which have definite shapes that lead to personification of the object and the projection onto it of human qualities. Secondary objects usually have a later onset, appearing in the second year of life or later and appear to be used to self-soothe and to deal with issues of autonomy and independence.

Secondary objects, such as teddy bears or family pets, have soothing qualities that provide the child with comfort, security, and companionship. They substitute for the mother when she is not available and are used when the child feels tense, tired, or ill (Triebenbacher, 1997). Children need little or no encouragement to self-soothe when anxious at bedtime or when meeting strangers by hugging, squeezing, or petting a stuffed animal. They also help develop autonomy since the small, inanimate doll is completely under the control of the child.

Texture appears to be a particularly important element of cuddly objects, even among nonhuman primates. You may recall that the classic research by Harry Harlow (Harlow & Zimmerman, 1958) found that isolated infant monkeys preferred contact with a soft cloth "mother" doll to contact with a wire "mother" doll that provided food. Typically, the infant monkeys would cling to the cloth doll about 22 hours a day.

By age 4 years, most "lovie"-attached children stop carrying their lovie, plush doll with them outside the home. However, many adolescents and adults never outgrow their attachment to cuddly toys. A recent survey of 6,000 adults by the Travelodge Hotel Company found that teddy bears accompany 35% of British adults to bed. The adults reported that the cuddly bears evoked a sense of peace, security, and comfort.

Rationale

Touching soft dolls produces feelings of pleasure and relaxation, which serve to counteract anxious and stressful affect. Also, plush dolls can serve as transitional objects that make us feel safe because they remind us of the softness and protection of a mother figure. According to Winnicott (1953), these transitional objects help children transition from a feeling of oneness with their mother to feelings of separateness and individuation.

Description

Ages

Two years and up.

Techniques

It is surprising that cuddly toys are not used more often in clinical practice. There is research support for the following applications:

Reducing Children's Discomfort in a Strange Situation, Like a Play Therapy Room

Passman and Weisberg (1975) found that when children were left in an unfamiliar playroom with a supportive agent such as a cuddly toy, the object enabled the children to play, explore, and refrain from crying more than a comparison group of children who had their favorite hard toy or who had no comforting object available.

Thus, it seems advisable to encourage children to bring their cuddly toys to their first play therapy sessions, or have several cuddly toys available for them in the playroom. You might ask the child to give the plush toy a name—for example, "Mrs. Huggabuggle"—the name given to a teddy bear by a 10-year-old girl in her first play therapy session.

Reducing Children's Distress in Stressful Situations, Such as Hospitalizations, Natural Disasters, Loss of a Loved One, Divorce

A growing number of studies have found that the practice of giving children a cuddly toy during stress times is beneficial in reducing their stress level.

Empirical Findings

1. In a study by Bloch and Taker (2008), a group of 41 preschool children were presented with a simulated hospital and asked to act as the parents of a teddy bear patient. Compared with a control group, the experimental group reported significantly lower levels of anxiety about future hospitalizations.

2. Epstein (2003, pp. 81–96) tells of a boy's attachment to a soft, sensitive plaything, a teddy bear. The 6-year-old boy entered the operating room clutching his teddy bear, which was then sent ahead to the recovery room after he was anesthetized. His surgery was long and traumatic—in fact, his heart stopped beating for an anguished 29 minutes midway through the surgery to open his spinal cord and remove a large, insidious tumor. When he awoke from the operation, the surgical team was relieved to see his brain function allowed the boy to inquire, "Who took my teddy bear?" as his first line of conversation.

3. Ullan and colleagues (2014) found in a randomized, controlled trial that when hospitalized young children (mean age of 3 years, 9 months; $n = 48$) were given a plush doll after undergoing surgery, their postsurgical pain was significantly reduced as compared with a control group. The doll was a plush toy rabbit, dressed as a doctor with a red cross on its chest. The authors attributed the results to the capacity of doll play to distract children and to improve their mood.

This plush doll was selected because in previous pilot studies, the researchers observed very good acceptance of this type of toy in hospitalized children. The children spontaneously displayed affectionate reactions toward this kind of doll (i.e., they hugged them, spoke to them, and were unwilling to be parted from them). The special "medical uniform" on the doll was selected because previous research (Burstein & Meichenbaum, 1979) reported evidence that when children played with toys that symbolically related to medical procedures just experienced, they tended to exhibit lower levels of anxiety in postoperative situations than children who did not play with such toys. It seems that play with these symbolic toys gives children a sense of control and mastery over a stressful medical experience they had no previous control over.

4. A study of psychiatrically hospitalized female adolescents (Jaffe & Franch, 1986) found that 12 of the 14 female adolescents had between one and 15 stuffed animals in their rooms. The girls appeared to use these treasured soft animals for comfort and security when fearful, to deal with separation anxiety, and for companionship.

5. In a study by Kushnir and Sadeh (2012), a group of 104 children ages 4–6 years suffering from severe nighttime fears were provided with a "huggy-puppy" intervention. Children in the experimental group were given a stuffed puppy toy and were asked to take care of the puppy or to view the doll as a protector or confidante to tell troubles to at bedtime. This randomized, controlled study found that, compared to a wait-list control group, the experimental children showed a significant reduction in nighttime fears—a major problem for preschool children. The gains were maintained at a 6-month follow-up.

6. Infants and toddlers who have "transitional objects" that they cling to at bedtime or when distressed have fewer sleep disturbances and are reported in three out of four studies to be more agreeable, self-confident, and affectionate (Litt, 1986).

Applications

Plush toys can serve as transitional objects to help young children cope with separations from their primary attachment figure. They can help relieve a shy, inhibited child's anxiety in social situations, and provide a source of comfort for children experiencing situational stress, such as hospitalization. Many adults also benefit from these comforting objects—for example, studies have found that plush toys, such as teddy bears, can improve the quality of life of patients with Alzheimer's disease by reducing agitation, distress, and withdrawal.

References

Ahluvalia, T., & Schaefer, C. E. (1994). Implications of transitional object use: A review of empirical findings. *Psychology, A Journal of Human Behavior, 31*(2), 45–57.

Bloch, Y., & Taker, A. (2008). Doctor, is my teddy bear OK?: The Teddy Bear Hospital as a method to reduce children's fear of hospitalization. *IMAJ: Israel Medical Association Journal, 10,* 597–599.

Bowlby, J. (1969). *Attachment and loss: Vol. 1. Attachment.* London: Hogarth Press.

Burstein, D., & Meichenbaum, D. (1979). The work of worrying in children undergoing surgery. *Journal of Abnormal Child Psychology, 7*(2), 121–132.

Epstein, F. (2003). *If I could get to five: What children can teach us about courage and character.* New York: Henry Holt.

Harlow, H., & Zimmerman, R. (1958). The development of affectional responses in infant monkeys. *Proceedings of the American Philosophical Society, 102*(5), 501–509.

Hong, K. (1978). The transitional phenomena. *Psychoanalytic Study of the Child, 3*, 47–79.

Jaffe, S., & Franch, K. (1986). The use of stuffed animals by hospitalized adolescents: An area for psychiatric exploration. *Journal of the American Academy of Child Psychiatry, 25*(4), 569–573.

Kushnir, J., & Sadeh, A. (2012). Assessment of brief interventions for nighttime fears in preschool children. *European Journal of Pediatrics, 171*, 67–75.

Litt, C. (1986). Theories of transitional object attachment: An overview. *International Journal of Behavioural Development, 9*, 383–399.

Passman, R., & Weisberg, P. (1975). Mothers and blankets as agents for promoting play and exploration by young children in a novel environment: The effects of social and non-social attachment objects. *Developmental Psychology, 11*, 170–177.

Triebenbacher, S. (1997). Children's use of transitional object: Parental attitudes and perceptions. *Child Psychology and Human Development, 27*(4), 221–230.

Ullan, A., Belver, M., Fernandez, E., Lorente, F., Badia, M., & Fernandez, B. (2014). The effect of a program to promote children's post-surgical pain: With plush toys, it hurts less. *Pain Management Nursing, 15*(1), 273–282.

Winnicott, D. W. (1953). Transitional objects and transitional phenomena. *International Journal of Psychoanalysis, 34*, 89–97.

Epilogue: Harlow's Wire Monkey Experiment

Harlow removed young monkeys a few hours after birth and left them to be raised by mother surrogates. The experiment revealed that the baby monkeys spent a great deal more time with their cloth mother than with their wire mother. He concluded that contact comfort is a variable of overwhelming importance in the development of affectionate responses, whereas lactation is a variable of much lesser importance.

The infant monkeys only went to wire monkeys when hungry. Once fed, they would return to the cloth mother for most of the day. If a frightening object was placed in their cage, they took refuge with the cloth mother.

(See the YouTube video "Harlow's Monkeys" [4:11 minutes; 2:07 to 2:32].)

3

Medical Play

Introduction

Medical play is a time-honored practice to help children cope with stressful medical experiences (e.g., doctor visits, hospitalization, dental check-ups). Nobody knows how long medical play goes back in time but it is probably as long as children have been treated by medical personnel.

Rationale

The therapeutic powers of play triggered by this technique include stress inoculation; catharsis, stress management; self-expression of anxieties/fears; and direct teaching of medical information and coping skills. Medical play can also provide a "working-through process" whereby children remember and repeat stressful medical experiences and gain mastery through the creation of positive outcomes where characters overcome illness and pain (Clark, 1998, 2003).

Description

Ages

Three years and up.

Materials

A pretend doctor's kit. Medical costumes are also recommended. Some specific medical play materials are:

- *Doctor Kit—Pretend Play Set (Meijer).* This doctor kit features enough medical tools for a whole team of young "doctors" to play at the same time. The sturdy plastic 19-piece set includes stethoscope and pager with realistic sounds, battery-operated cellphone, forceps, bandages thermometer, and more. Everything fits into a handy (12 × 14 × 3½ inches) plastic clamp-tight case. Batteries for stethoscope and pager included.

• *Doctor Role Play Costume Set (Melissa & Doug)*. Contains doctor costumes, face masks, stethoscope with sound effects, reflex hammer, ear scope, and syringe. Playmobil has a line of *pretend medical settings* (operating room, dentist's office, etc.) with appropriate toy figures. They are hard plastic so they can be washed or wiped after each use.

It is best to supplement pretend doctor kits with real medical equipment, such as needleless syringes, stethoscopes, gauze, Band-Aids, intravenous tubing, tape, and unbreakable thermometers.

Techniques

Role Reversal

The child role-plays a doctor/nurse performing an exam or procedure on a therapist, doctor, nurse, pet, or a play object (e.g., stuffed animal). This is often enacted *after* a child has experienced an anxiety-provoking medical procedure. It gives the child a sense of power and control over a stressful event in which he/she felt helpless and powerless. Children often pretend to be a doctor, nurse, or child life specialist "teaching their dolls, stuffed animals, or family members what to expect during a medical treatment." In this way, they gain a sense of mastery over the experience.

Stress Inoculation Role Play

A therapist or parent plays the role of a doctor performing a medical procedure on a patient (child, puppet, or doll patient). This role play helps the child become familiar with an upcoming, stressful procedure, learn skills to cope with the procedure, and express fears, anxieties, and misperceptions about the medical experience.

Empirical Findings

1. After reviewing the empirical support for play therapy, Phillips (2010) concluded that the most compelling evidence for play therapy's effectiveness is found for children facing medical procedures.

2. More specifically, Zahr (1998) presented a puppet show to 50 preschoolers the day before their scheduled surgery. Puppets representing the child, the parents, a doctor, and a nurse played out the sequence of medical events the child would experience, from admission to discharge, with an explanation about what to expect and what sensations would be felt. The children were allowed to play with the puppets, handle the medical objects, and reenact the play. Compared with a control group that received routine care but no therapeutic play, the experimental group manifested markedly less anxiety and more cooperation and had significantly lower mean blood pressures and pulse rates during injections.

3. Nabors and colleagues (2013) conducted an investigation of the use of medical play as a coping mechanism for children undergoing hospital medical procedures and their siblings. The children ranged in age from 2 to 10 years. The results indicated that the children with chronic illnesses and their siblings gravitated toward and benefited from expressing and releasing their feelings while engaged in unstructured medical play where they replayed negative medical procedures. The medical play produced a sense of mastery, as most characters became healthy again. In contrast, children in the control group did not engage in much medical play.

Applications

Medical play is appropriate for children exhibiting fears or anxieties about forthcoming or recently experienced medical procedures, including hospitalized children and children facing visits to a doctor's office. In many cases, a child's medical care can have a strong impact on his/her siblings and produce medical anxiety in them as well. Often the siblings will want to engage in medical play so that they too can receive special attention from their parents.

Contraindications

Medical play may trigger intense anxiety in a child who had undergone a very traumatic medical experience.

References

Clark, C. D. (1998). Childhood imagination in the face of chronic illness. In J. de Rivera & T. R. Sarbin (Eds.), *Believed-in imaginings: The narrative construction of reality* (pp. 87–100). Washington, DC: American Psychological Association.

Clark, C. D. (2003). *In sickness and in play: Children coping with chronic illness.* Brunswick, NJ: Rutgers University Press.

Nabors, L., Bartz, J., Kichler, J., Sievers, R., Elkins, R., & Pangello, J. (2013). Play as a mechanism of working through medical trauma for children with medical illnesses and their siblings. *Issues in Comprehensive Pediatric Nursing, 36*(3), 212–224.

Phillips, R. (2010). How firm is our foundation?: Current play therapy research. *International Journal of Play Therapy, 19*(1), 13–25.

Zahr, L. (1998). Therapeutic play for hospitalized preschoolers in Lebanon. *Pediatric Nursing, 23*(5), 449–454.

4

Baby Doll Play

Introduction

Children, ages 2 years and up, have played with dolls since the beginning of civilization. Evidence exists that dolls were part of Greek and Roman life and wooden and clay dolls were found in Egyptian temples. European dolls, which most closely resemble the playthings of today, debuted in the 14th century in Germany.

Rationale

• Baby doll play provides an outlet for the child's expression of conscious and unconscious material. Baby dolls give children an object that they can use to project their feelings about babies and family relationships. Dolls also allow children to reenact real-life traumatic events, such as abuse/neglect, and to ask for nurturance for themselves—for example, a 6-year-old girl who enacts a scene wherein a mother doll beats the baby doll severely for wetting the bed and threatens to "kill her" is likely expressing important clinical information about her abuse at home (Cattanach, 1993).

• Play with baby dolls provides an opportunity to practice nurturing and caring for others. A therapist playing with a baby doll can model nurturing behaviors for a young child.

• Such play can help prepare children for the addition of a new baby. For instance, baby doll play by an adult can model for children how to care for a baby (e.g., how to hold, handle, act, and speak around a newborn).

• Baby dolls can provide comfort and security for children (i.e., use the soft doll as a transitional, security object).

• Taking care of a doll can foster a sense of competence in a child. Assuming an adult role fosters a sense of power and control for young children who have very little control over their world.

• A corrective emotional experience is also possible though baby doll play. For an abused/neglected child, one can model giving the baby doll the loving care the child did not receive in real life. Since the child will likely identify with the doll, the child will indirectly receive the nurturance.

Description

Ages

Two years and up.

Materials

A large assortment of realistic, high-quality baby dolls (14–19 inches tall) are commercially available for both girls and boys. By around 2 or 3 years old children typically begin to act as if their doll can see and interact with them. Choose dolls that are soft, washable, and made of nontoxic material.

Interactive dolls that require empathic responding (e.g., eats, wets, cries) are a great asset for teaching and practicing nurturing and caring for others (social–emotional skills) because the child needs to respond to the baby's signals.

Examples of commercially available baby dolls are Interactive Baby Annabelle Doll (Zapf) and Baby Alive (Hasbro).

Technique

Nurturing Role Play

This technique can be useful when a child is mistreating a baby doll or he/she was mistreated as a baby. During baby doll play the therapist consistently acts as a nurturing role model—for example, the therapist displays and handles the doll with great care as a real baby would be cared for, in a loving way. A baby doll is not an ordinary toy. It represents a child, so it needs to have its own name and be introduced to the child. It is best to have lots of props available, such as a bottle, baby food, dishes and spoons for feeding, a crib for sleeping, nighttime and daytime clothes, diapers, and so on.

If a child is mistreating a doll, provide empathy for the doll, interrupt serious maltreatment, and try to explain why the baby is acting the way it is. If a child cannot take care of the doll, put it away in your care until the child can take proper care of it.

Empirical Findings

Baby dolls have been used therapeutically with increasing frequency with adults suffering from severe dementia. Tamura, Kakajima, and Nambu (2001) found that it tends to comfort them; calm/reduce agitation; facilitate communication; and generates warm, nurturing feelings that makes these adults happier.

Applications

This technique is particularly useful for children who present with attachment issues related to adoption, histories of abuse and/or neglect during infancy, and other early losses and separations. It is also appropriate for children who are aggressive at home, because the doll provides a safe outlet for the child to displace angry feelings toward parents or siblings.

References

Cattanach, A. (1993). *Play therapy with abused children*. London; Jessica Kingsley.
Tamura, T., Kakajima, K., & Nambu, M. (2001). Baby dolls as therapeutic tools for severe dementia patients. *Gerontechnology, 1*(2), 111–118.

5

Baby Bottle Play

Introduction

In his theory of personality development, Sigmund Freud (1953) proposed that infants derive pleasure from the act of sucking and learn to love from the mother who rocks, kisses, and cuddles during feedings. Eric Erickson (1963) proposed that the infant's experiences during this first stage of life result in a sense of basic trust or mistrust toward self and others. Based on these theories and research related to attachment behavior, the baby bottle has significant psychological meaning and is a powerful tool for accessing and treating children's needs and feelings associated with nurturance and soothing. This is illustrated in a clinical vignette described by Anna Freud (1964):

> When the group went into the playroom, the boys, with the exception of Buddy, made a dash for the nursing bottles and began sucking them. Charles picked up the toy telephone.
>
> CHARLES: I'm going to call my mother. She works at _____. I want to talk to her.
> THERAPIST: You would like to talk to your mother.
> CHARLES: Hello, Mother. I'm just a baby, Mother. (*Sucks on bottle*.) I'm taking my bottle now. You better come home.
> THERAPIST: You want your mother to come home and take care of her baby. (p. 229)

Rationale

Axline (1947) and Moustakas (1979) listed baby bottles as one of the most important toys for play therapy. Baby bottles provide several therapeutic benefits. These include:

• *Communication.* Baby bottles provide a way for children to express conscious, subconscious, and drive-related feelings and needs. Murray (1997) wrote:

> One disturbed boy initially would rarely answer me when I spoke to him, but would suck water out of the bottle. It was the only way he took away from the session any good feelings for a while. It seemed to serve as a bridge between us. (p. 238)

• *Addressing unmet needs.* Baby bottles are particularly helpful for children who present with unmet needs for nurturance. Bowlby (1969) proposed that infants develop an "internal working model" based on their relationship with the primary caregiver. This model is an internalized understanding of self, the world, and the way relationships work. According to this theory, memories, experiences, and expectations from the child's internal model have a significant effect on his/ her sense of self and interactions with others. Benedict and Mongoven (1997) note that children with histories of traumatic, painful, or neglectful parenting develop negative working models. The goal of treatment is to help them see relationships as giving, nurturing, and safe. Benedict and Mongoven wrote:

> The therapist may take on the role of a caregiver and provide nurturance to the child as if he/she were an infant. The therapist may feed, hold, rock, or read to him/her as a way to provide the nurturance that he/she needs. (p. 301)

• *Attachment formation.* Use of the baby bottle in treatment can foster a sense of trust and attachment. Benedict and Mongoven (1997) note that the therapist's sensitivity to the child's needs can help to engage him/her in treatment and foster a trusting relationship. This is illustrated in the following case:

> She walked into the therapy room, appearing rather drowsy, and started to play with the therapist's dolls. She hugged them, kissed them, and used bottles to feed them. The feeding ritual continued for quite some time; it appeared that the "babies" were very hungry. After feeding the dolls, Maria took one of the bottles and pretended to feed herself. The therapist recognized Maria's interest in the bottle and offered her a larger bottle "of her very own." Maria appeared very excited and immediately began to suck on her bottle vigorously. (Benedict & Mongoven, 1997, p. 307)

• *Comfort and soothing.* Children who suck on baby bottles in play therapy often smile and wear expressions of pleasure. Murray (1997) wrote:

> These children lie down and suck and smile. The smile is one of pleasure and seems also one of secret collaboration, as if they're thinking, "I know I'm too old for this but it's fun and I'm glad you're letting me do this." (p. 238)

• *Fantasy.* "Pretending gives a child power over the world" (Schaefer, 1993, p. 10). However, children with early experiences of emotional isolation and abuse often lack the development of symbolic play.

• *Mastery.* Using a baby bottle to encourage regressive infant-type play allows children to work through and master fears and anxieties based on unmet needs (Holmberg & Benedict, n.d.; Schaefer, 1997).

Description

Ages

Three to 6 years.

Materials

Plastic baby bottle or sports bottle filled with water.

Techniques

For young children who have displayed a need for nurturance, provide a baby bottle in the play room. Each child using the bottle should have his/her own for sanitary reasons. Baby bottles are most commonly used in a nondirective way where the child takes the lead. The therapist then addresses feelings and needs that are expressed in the play. However, Schaefer (1997) introduced a structured technique for parents called the "playing baby game." This technique was developed to address the emotional needs of young children following the birth of a sibling. In this activity, the mother sets aside a special place and time each day to play with the child as if he/she were a baby again. Baby bottles, blankets, and other baby toys are used to encourage regression and a sense of nurturance and security. This technique reduces feelings of rivalry and resentment of children who are struggling with having a new sibling.

Variation

The nurturing play techniques of Theraplay (Booth & Jernberg, 2009) are designed to model for parents how to foster a secure attachment in their child.

Empirical Findings

1. Lebo (1979) examined the number of statements made while children used particular toys during therapy. She then converted this number into a "verbal index." The baby (nursing) bottle was determined to be one of the top 28 toys that offer a "quantity and variety" of statements.

2. Ryan (1999) used the baby bottle to help a developmentally delayed child understand and become engaged in symbolic play. Ryan reported the following case example:

Patrick has the therapist help him unscrew the bottle, then he asks her if she wants a drink, saying he is too big.

T: I don't mind. If you want me to.

Patrick has the therapist screw the top back on after he fills the bottle with orange drink by himself.

P: You drink it.
T: All right. Maybe I'm a baby?
P: Yeah.
T: Waah! Where's my bottle?

Patrick smiles slightly and gives the therapist the bottle to drink. She drinks it, making satisfied noises (*Mmmmmm*) while she drinks. Patrick watches very intently, but without any sign of enjoyment at the therapist's pretend play. The therapist finishes sucking the bottle after a short time.

T: (*smiling*) It's very odd to see a big lady drinking a bottle.

She drinks a bit more while Patrick stares intently.

P: Want some more?
T: I can. I don't really drink out of a bottle, do I? I'm just playing I'm drinking out of a bottle now.

Patrick then starts pretending, although very unsurely, that he is taking the caregiver's role, telling the therapist to wait while he refills the bottle, managing to unscrew and screw it again himself. He gives the therapist a lot more to drink.

P: Drink it.
T: (*smiling*) You're taking care of me, giving me lots of drinks. (p. 174)

Applications

Baby bottles are especially useful for treating children with histories of loss, abuse, separation, insecure attachment, and trauma. Baby bottles are also helpful for children adjusting to the birth of a new sibling and other environmental challenges that bring up feelings of loss and insecurity.

Contraindications

Nurturing play is not appropriate for children who are not comfortable regressing to a dependent, helpless state, or when parents are wary or opposed to play that promotes regression in their child.

References

Axline, V. M. (1947). *Play therapy: The inner dynamics of childhood.* Oxford, UK: Houghton Mifflin.

Benedict, H. E., & Mongoven, L. B. (1997). Thematic play therapy: An approach to treatment of attachment disorders in young children. In H. G. Kaduson, D. Cangelosi, & C. Schaefer (Eds.), *The playing cure* (pp. 277–315). Northvale, NJ: Jason Aronson.

Booth, P., & Jernberg, A. (2009). *Theraplay: Helping parents and children build better relationships through attachment-based play* (3rd ed.). San Francisco: Jossey-Bass.

Bowlby, J. (1969). *Attachment and loss: Vol. 1. Attachment.* London: Hogarth Press.

Erikson, E. H. (1963). *Childhood and society.* Middlesex, UK: Penguin Books.

Freud, A. (1964). *The psychoanalytic treatment of children.* New York: International Universities Press.

Freud, S. (1953). Three essays on the theory of sexuality. *Standard Edition, 7,* 125–245.

Holmberg, J. R., & Benedict, H. (n.d.). Play therapy: How does that work anyway?: A resource handout for parents. Retrieved from *www.gapt.org/pdf_files/ARTICLES%20VOL%20 1-9/08-01%20(2)%20PT%20HOW%20DOES%20THAT%20WORK-HOLM-BERG.pdf.*

Lebo, D. (1979). Toys for nondirective play therapy. In C. E. Schaefer (Ed.), *Therapeutic use of child's play* (pp. 435–447). New York: Jason Aronson.

Moustakas, C. E. (1979). *Psychotherapy with children: The living relationship.* Oxford, UK: Harper.

Murray, D. (1997). The baby bottle technique. In H. G. Kaduson & C. E. Schaefer (Eds.), *101 favorite play therapy techniques* (pp. 236–238). Northvale, NJ: Jason Aronson.

Ryan, V. (1999). Developmental delay, symbolic play and non-directive play therapy. *Clinical Child Psychology and Psychiatry, 4*(2), 167–185.

Schaefer, C. E. (1993). *The therapeutic powers of play.* Northvale, NJ: Jason Aronson.

Schaefer, C. E. (1997). The playing baby technique. In H. G. Kaduson & C. E. Schaefer (Eds.), *101 favorite play therapy techniques* (pp. 3–5). Northvale, NJ: Jason Aronson.

Toy Telephone Play

Introduction

Beginning at ages 3–4 years children show the ability to engage in real-life telephone conversations (Gillen, 2002). They also play with toy telephones and find this play a useful way to communicate indirectly with the therapist or with someone else they are not ready or able to speak with directly. The phones can be used to tell what they really feel but choose not to say, to verbalize what they wish they had been able to say, or to rehearse what needs to be said. Play therapists have used the pretend phone play technique with children and adolescents for over 75 years (Durfee, 1942).

Rationale

- *Facilitates self-expression.* Pretending to talk on a toy telephone can give a child who is reluctant to talk or maintain eye contact enough psychological distance to engage in a conversation with the therapist or an imaginary person.
- *Ego boosting.* The use of a telephone tends to be perceived by young children as a source of power, control, maturity, and accomplishment.

Description

Ages

Four to 12 years.

Materials

Two toy cellphones or two old, disabled real phones.

Techniques

Therapist–Child Phone Conversation

By answering the therapist's questions indirectly on the phone, a child may be able to express what he/she finds too difficult to say face-to-face. If the phone talk is too difficult, the child can just hang up. The therapist might ask the child about his/her day—that is, the activities or feelings experienced, or whatever the child wants to talk about. This simple technique can make the child feel special and can jump-start a conversation with a quiet child.

Imaginary Conversation

Pretend phone play can encourage a child to have a two-way conversation with an absent, deceased, or imaginary person. By age 7 years, children are generally able to play the role of both sender and receiver of a phone message. This pretend conversation can reveal a great deal about a child's real or desired social interactions.

The therapist might suggest that the child do one or more of the following role-play phone conversations:

"Pretend to call home."
"Pretend to call a deceased or absent parent."
"Pretend to call a friend you had when you were younger."
"Pretend to call yourself as a child."
"Pretend you are your mother and call me and ask how you are doing."
"Pretend to call God or the good fairy and ask that a wish come true."
"Pretend to call your stomach (or other body part) and ask why it is hurting."
"Pretend to call your teacher."
"Pretend to call the wise person inside of you for advice."
"Pretend to call the monster in your bad dream."

Alternatively, the therapist can pretend receiving phone calls from the above (e.g., "Ring, ring. Hello, yes he is here. Peter, your mommy wants to talk with you!").

Broadcast News

In this technique (Hall, Kaduson, & Schaefer, 2002), the child and therapist pretend to be delivering a radio news broadcast to other children who call in and ask questions that the child as the expert on the topic will answer, such as coping with ADD. The therapist plays the role of the telephone callers, which provides the opportunity to highlight the child's accomplishments and ongoing issues in therapy. The child may gain self-confidence by discovering problem-solving abilities and resources through this role-play activity.

Case Illustration

Spero (1980) reported the case of an abused 8-year-old girl who had great difficulty accepting her negative feelings toward her violent mother. Her descriptions of her mother were of a pleasant, well-intentioned, and nurturing person. Early in therapy, her therapist suggested that she call her mother at home on the toy phone to ask if she could be picked up from school early. Acting in the role of her mother, the girl said that having her home would be "inconvenient and would upset her day." When the girl asked a second time, complaining of a headache, her mother stated that she would be punished for messing up the daily schedule. Although the girl could not confront and accept her negative image of her mother directly, she fantasized a typical interchange between them.

Empirical Findings

Gillen and Hall (2001) found that pretend telephone play increased the social communication skills of 3- and 4-year-old children.

Applications

Telephone play is particularly helpful for shy, inhibited children who have difficulty expressing themselves with strangers. It offers these children a safe psychological distance to express their inner world of thoughts, feelings, and desires.

References

Durfee, M. (1942). Use of ordinary office equipment in play therapy. *American Journal of Orthopsychiatry*, 2, 495–502.

Gillen, J. (2002). Moves in the territory of literacy?: The telephone discourses of three-and four-year-olds. *Journal of Early Childhood Literacy*, 2(1), 21–43.

Gillen, J., & Hall, N. (2001). "Hiya, Mum!": An analysis of pretence telephone play in a nursery setting. *Early Years: An International Research Journal*, 21(1), 15–24.

Hall, T., Kaduson, H., & Schaefer, C. (2002). Fifteen effective play therapy techniques. *Professional Psychology: Research and Practice*, 33(6), 515–522.

Spero, M. (1980). Use of the telephone in child play therapy. *Social Work*, 25(1), 57–60.

7

Magic Wand Play

Introduction

A magic wand is a stick-like object purported to have magic powers. Magic wands date back to ancient Egypt where wands were placed in the tombs of pharaohs so their soul could use them. The earliest magic wand in Western literature appears in the *Odyssey*—the enchantress Circe uses it to transform Odysseus's men into swine. Most recently, personal wands were the common tool of the wizards in J. K. Rowling's *Harry Potter* novels.

In regard to developmental changes in the "three wishes" technique, Ables (1972) found that children in grades 3 through 6 most commonly wished for material things. Other common wishes were for another person, such as a sibling; specific personal skills or attributes; pets; an activity; money; and more wishes.

The most common wishes of college students (King & Broyles, 1997) were for friends, happiness, health, marriage, money, success, self-improvement, and to help other people. Although men's and women's wishes were generally similar, men were more likely to wish for sex and power, and women were more likely to wish for happiness, a better appearance, and improved health. Horrocks and Mussman (1973) discovered that as children mature into adulthood their wishes become more general and altruistic and less materialistic. In addition, a gradual increase in achievement wishes was evident through middle adulthood.

Rationale

This reality therapy technique was introduced by the psychiatrist William Glasser (1965), who believed that the client will identify the actual issue at hand when making three personalized wishes. One of these wishes will be the actual problem or issue the child is facing. Typically, the client will disclose unmet needs and desires, which then can be discussed in order to set realistic goals for therapy.

28

Description

Ages

Four years and up.

Materials

The wand can be anything from a brightly decorated purchased wand, or a uniquely shaped stick.

Technique

Three Wishes

This technique involves showing a child a magic wand and saying, "Imagine that with a wave of this magic wand I could make three of your wishes come true. What would you wish for? An alternate instruction is "Imagine that with a wave of this wand you could change anything in your life or in the world. What would you change?"

Variations

Special Power Wands

Show the child wands with specific powers—for example, one wand can make your wish to change anything you want about yourself come true, or you could change anything you want about your family (Allen, 2003). A second wand can make another person change his/her behavior. A third can obtain any material thing you desire. Discuss with the child how life would be better with such changes, and how to set goals for needed changes.

Miracle Question

In solution-focused therapy (Miller, 1996), the "miracle question" can make a client's wish for a future goal more specific. The therapist initiates this technique by saying, "Imagine that when you fall asleep tonight a miracle happened—almost as if a magic wand waved over you and the problem or difficulty you are currently experiencing is eliminated. You are not aware of what has happened when you were sleeping, but you notice the changes. What is it you notice when you wake up, and as you continue through your day, that lets you know that a miracle has occurred?"

A similar question that is often asked by Adlerian play therapists is "If this magic wand would eliminate your problem immediately, what would be different in your life?"

Magic Key

In this technique (Crenshaw, 2005), the therapist asks the child to imagine that he/ she has been given a magic key to a room in a castle that contains the one thing missing from his/her life or the one thing that would increase happiness. After visualizing the thing in the room, the child is asked to draw a picture of it.

Wizard Wands

Popescu and Gane (2011) developed a "wizarding" psychotherapy program for children ages 6–12 years that integrates the magic wand technique into the program. The Harry Potter–type wand is used as a problem-solving strategy, as well as a safety and attachment object for the child.

Magic Carpet

Place a colorful, fringed carpet in the playroom and invite the child to sit on it and imagine that it has the power to transport him/her to faraway places, escape an unpleasant situation, or simply for use as a safe place of peace or solitude (Conyers, 1997).

Magic Box

Ask the child to pretend that you have put a magic box on the table in from of him/ her. The magic box contains anything the child wishes. Ask the child to open the box and tell you what is inside. The goal is to reveal deep wishes and desires that are in the child's psyche.

Magic Tricks

The mystery, excitement, and challenge of a few magic tricks performed by a therapist are likely to capture the interest of school-age children. Magic can help establish initial rapport with them (Gilroy, 1998) and overcome resistance to therapy (Bow, 1988). It is best to use simple magic tricks that children can learn and try for themselves. (See Chapter 55, "Magic Tricks," for further elaboration of this procedure.)

Three Wishes for My Family

Developed by family play therapist Katherine Arkell, this technique consists of presenting each member of a family with a clipboard containing three sheets of paper and asking them to draw three wishes for their family—one wish on each sheet. They may draw whatever they want but may not use any letters or words. Then the members share their drawings by holding them up for the others to guess what the wishes are.

Empirical Findings

The magic wand technique is in need of empirical research.

Applications

Magic wand play can help all child clients express their unmet needs and hidden wishes. This can serve as a springboard for a discussion of realistic ways to satisfy those needs and desires that underlie their presenting problem.

References

Ables, A. (1972). The three wishes of latency age children. *Developmental Psychology*, 6(1), 186.

Allen, V. (2003). The magic wand. In H. G. Kaduson & C. E. Schaefer (Eds.), *101 favorite play therapy techniques* (Vol. 3, pp. 303–305). Northvale, NJ: Jason Aronson.

Bow, J. N. (1988). Treating resistant children. *Child and Adolescent Social Work*, 5, 3–15.

Conyers, D. (1997). The magic carpet technique. In H. Kaduson & C. Schaefer (Eds.), *101 favorite play therapy techniques* (pp. 230–232). Northvale, NJ: Jason Aronson.

Crenshaw, D. (2005). Clinical tools to facilitate treatment of traumatic grief. *Omega: Journal of Death and Dying, 51*, 239–255.

Gilroy, B. D. (1998). *Counseling kids: It's magic, therapeutic uses of magic with children and teens*. Scotch Plains, NJ: Therapist Organizer.

Glasser, W. D. (1965). *Reality therapy: A new approach to psychiatry*. New York: Harper & Row.

Horrocks, J., & Mussman, M. (1973). Developmental trends in wishes, confidence, and sense of personal control from childhood to middle maturity. *Journal of Psychology: Interdisciplinary and Applied, 84*(2), 241–252.

King, L. A., & Broyles, S. J. (1997). Wishes, gender, personality, and well-being. *Journal of Personality, 65*, 49–76.

Miller, S. (1996). *Handbook of solution-focused brief therapy*. San Francisco: Jossey-Bass.

Popescu, O., & Gane, S. (2011). The wizarding school: A psychotherapy program for children. *International Journal of Integrative Psychotherapy, 2*(2), 1–18.

8

Bubble Play

Introduction

Children have played with soap bubbles since at least the 17th century when paintings depicting this kind of play appeared in what is now modern-day Belgium. The more than 200 million bottles of bubbles sold annually attest to its continuing popularity. Bubbles are made of air trapped inside a hollow liquid ball. The colors visible in bubbles come from light reflected in the bubble's surface. Bubbles float up because warm air is lighter than cold air. If the air blown into the bubble is warmer than the air around it, the bubble will float up.

Rationale

Among the therapeutic benefits of bubble blowing for children are mood elevation, rapport building, modeling therapeutic breathing, distraction during a stressful event, and group cohesion.

Description

Ages

Three to 6 years.

Materials

Bottle of bubble liquid and a bubble wand.

Techniques

Bubble Breaths

Young children love to blow bubbles and they can use this activity to learn deep breathing to relax themselves. First, ask the child to hold up the wand and blow quickly. The result will be a lot of small bubbles. Then ask the child to take a deep breath and blow slowly (for about 4 seconds). This should result in fewer but bigger bubbles. Model this for the child. The long breaths needed for blowing large bubbles are identical to the breaths needed for relaxation breathing. Point out to the child that this bubble-blowing activity is to learn how to relax when he/she is feeling anxious. This is a tool the child can use anytime.

"Fun" Bubble Play

The fun of blowing, chasing, catching, and popping bubbles can lift a child's spirits and promote bonding among preschool children. This is helpful for children under stress and children with social difficulties.

Empirical Findings

Chilamakuri, Nuvvula, and Sunkara (2014) report from their experience in pediatric dentistry that the bubble breath procedure is a simple, engaging, yet highly effective technique for teaching a concrete relaxation method for children in the stressful situations involving dental work.

Applications

Bubble breaths is an excellent way to teach children to relax and calm themselves when they are emotionally upset or experiencing a stressful situation, such as a medical procedure or injection.

References

Chilamakuri, S., Nuvvula, S., & Sunkara, N. (2014). Play therapy in pediatric dentistry. *Journal of Pediatric Dentistry, 2*(1), 28.

9

Block Play

Introduction

The urge to construct objects with blocks is evident early in life and is a universal human tendency. For over 100 years blocks have been considered the most useful, durable, and versatile toy in early childhood classrooms. In addition to building with blocks, Lincoln Logs, Legos, and Tinkertoys have been popular alternatives for children. In addition to building with blocks, knocking down a tower of blocks is a fun activity for young children (Hanline, 2001).

Rationale

Therapists have used block play to increase children's cognitive development by asking them to engage in an activity that requires planning ahead and anticipating the consequences of one's actions (Cartwright, 1974), to promote their social development by asking a family or peer group to build a house or other object together (Rogers, 1987), to elevate their mood by participating in an enjoyable and challenging activity, to foster the catharsis of aggression by having them knock down a block construction, and to boost their egos by strengthening their problem-solving ability and sense of competence.

Description

Ages

Three years and up.

Materials

For preschool children ages 3–5 years, a set of large cardboard blocks, foam or hollow wood blocks, or Duplo blocks are developmentally appropriate. For older children, solid wood unit blocks are popular. The smooth, sanded surface; precise mathematical proportions; and endless building possibilities make unit blocks appealing to all children. School-age children and adolescents also enjoy assembling Lego blocks. These little plastic Lego blocks made their debut in the 1940s. Lego was named "Toy of the Century" in 2000 by *Fortune* magazine as well as the British Toy Retailers Association.

Techniques

Dyadic Tutoring

The therapist acts as a block play tutor—instructing, modeling, prompting, and reinforcing cooperation during interactive construction play with a child lacking social skills.

Group Construction

One activity or teaching social skills to a group of children ages 4–8 years is to involve them in a group play with blocks. Short (1997) recommends presenting children with a big basket of wood blocks (all sizes and colors) and asking them to build something together. There are just two rules. First, they must use all the blocks, and second is that everyone must be allowed to help. The goal is to foster cooperation, teamwork, and cohesiveness.

Family Block Play

Present the family with a large box of building blocks and ask them to make something with the blocks, such as a house. The therapist observes family interaction patterns (e.g., alliances, leadership, noninvolved members).

Knocking Down the Walls of Anger

In this technique (Leonetti, 1997), a child throws a rubber ball to topple a wall of hollow or cardboard blocks while stating something that makes him/her angry. The goal is to provide a cathartic release of anger for children who have difficulty expressing their emotions.

"Don't Break the Ice" Game

Children find the commercial Don't Break the Ice game to be fun, challenging, and exciting. It can be used therapeutically to establish rapport or provide a cathartic release of feelings (Cangelosi, 1997). One application of this game is to ask the child to describe a situation that caused him/her to feel angry, frustrated, hurt, sad, or mad. The child then taps out a block of ice with the plastic mallet to "get rid of the feeling." The therapist prompts the child to think about ways to effectively handle the situation in the future. The therapist then takes a turn to model effective coping to get rid of a personal negative feeling. The therapist and child continue to take turns until all the ice blocks have been tapped away.

Alternately, Kenny-Noziska (2008) has used the Don't Break the Ice game with latency-age children to establish rapport. When the child or therapist taps out a block of ice, he/she has to say something about him/herself—for example, a favorite food or TV show.

Jenga

The word *jenga* is derived from the Swahili word meaning "to build." The game was created in the 1970s by Leslie Scott, a British National, and is currently distributed by Parker Brothers. This is a stacking game for two or more players ages 6 years and up. Initially, the 54 wooden blocks are used to build a tower (18 levels of three blocks each). The first player then uses one hand to take a block from any level and place it on top of the stack—without toppling the stack (or any block from it). The game fosters concentration, problem solving, and frustration tolerance. The playing time is usually 5–15 minutes.

Lego Therapy

The Lego system of blocks and other objects is a structured, predictable, and systematic construction toy. It is therefore not surprising that children with autism spectrum disorder (ASD) are motivated by tasks involving this toy because individuals with this condition are particularly attracted to systems. Children participating in Lego therapy (Legoff, 2004) first learn a set of clear "Lego Club" rules and develop Lego brick-building skills, including collaborative building, in individual therapy. In the group-therapy sessions, the children learn to communicate with others, express feelings, modify troublesome behavior, develop problem-solving skills, and a variety of ways of relating positively to others. Lego-based interactive play groups have been found effective in improving the social skills of children and adolescents, especially those with ASDs (Legoff & Sherman, 2006).

Empirical Findings

1. Rogers (1985) observed that during block play with peers, kindergarten children exhibited prosocial behaviors, such as smiling, taking turns, helping, and asking (as opposed to commanding) three times more frequently than antisocial behaviors, such as hitting and throwing blocks.

2. Legoff and Sherman (2006) reported that children with autism who are high functioning, ages 8–12 years, and received group Lego therapy improved significantly more in social competence than children in the control group.

Applications

Play with building materials promotes self-control because it requires planning ahead, impulse control, and frustration tolerance. Thus, it is particularly useful for children with ADD and ADHD. It has also been found effective in promoting cooperative play in preschool and school-age children, as well as with children and adolescents with autism who are high functioning.

References

Cangelosi, D. (1997). Pounding away bad feelings. In H. G. Kaduson & C. E. Schaefer (Eds.), *101 favorite play therapy techniques* (pp. 142–144). Northvale, NJ: Jason Aronson.

Cartwright, S. (1974). Blocks and learning. *Young Children, 15*, 141–146.

Hanline, N. (2001). Young children's block construction activity. *Journal of Early Intervention, 24*(3), 224–237.

Kenny-Noziska, S. (2008). *Techniques–techniques–techniques. Play-based activities for children, adolescents, and families.* West Conskohocken, PA: Infinity.

Legoff, D. (2004). Use of Lego as a therapeutic medium for improving social competence. *Journal of Autism and Developmental Disorders, 34*(5), 587–598.

Legoff, D., & Sherman, M. (2006). Long-term outcome of social skills intervention based on interactive LEGO play. *Autism, 10*(4), 317–329.

Leonetti, J. (1997). Knocking down the walls of anger. In H. G. Kaduson & C. E. Schaefer (Eds.), *101 favorite play therapy techniques* (pp. 286–290). Northvale, NJ: Jason Aronson.

Rogers, D. (1987, Spring). Fostering social development through block play. *Day Care and Early Education*, pp. 26–29.

Rogers, D. L. (1985). Relationship between block play and the social development of young children. *Early Child Development and Care, 20*, 245–261.

Short, G. (1997). Group building activity. In H. G. Kaduson & C. E. Schaefer (Eds.). *101 favorite play therapy techniques* (pp. 299–300). Northvale, NJ: Jason Aronson.

10

Balloon Play

Introduction

Balloons were invented in the mid-1800s by Michael Faraday, but it was not until 1931 that there was mass production of modern-day self-blow-up colored, latex balloons (Swain, 2010). Since that time, balloon play has proven to be an extremely popular activity that has been enjoyed by countless children. They have found many ways to have fun with balloons, such as juggling, swatting, popping, painting, and bouncing them.

Rationale

Balloon play has been used to foster the catharsis of aggression, assertiveness, and the development of metaphorical insight into ways to relax and calm down one's level of arousal and stress.

Description

Ages

Three years and up.

Materials

An assortment of round (9–12 inches), colorful latex balloons. Balloons work best for games when blown up at about 85% of inflation capacity.

Techniques

Balloon Bursting

Balloon bursting was first used by Levy (1938) in his structured "release therapy" approach. The primary purpose of his simple strategy was to promote assertiveness in timid, inhibited, or fearful children (ages 3–8 years) by bursting balloons and thereby releasing suppressed aggressive energy. The therapist provides a number of colorful balloons of assorted sizes and shapes and says, "Now let's play with balloons!" It is very important that the first balloon be blown up only a little bit, so that when it breaks it does not make such a loud noise that the child is frightened and stops playing. The therapist then encourages the child to break the balloon in any way he/she pleases. Stamping and jumping are most common. Special tools—nails, mallets, dart guns, and so on—should be available to the child for playing out specific problems or impulses. As the play progresses, more balloons are provided that are closer to the bursting point. With very anxious children, it may be necessary to precede this balloon play with less startling forms of noise making, such as paper rattling, shouting, and so on. After a balloon-popping activity, the therapist helps the child process the positive feelings experienced during the activity (e.g., powerfulness, assertiveness, bravery).

Anger Release

First discuss with the child various coping mechanisms for reducing angry feelings, such as bubble breaths (slow, deep breathing), talking, and stomping feet. Then while blowing up and tying off a balloon, mention how sometimes kids can get so angry they feel like they will explode. Demonstrate an explosion by asking the child to stomp on or burst the balloon with a pin. Blow up another balloon and give it to the child to hold closed by its end. Then mention a coping mechanism and ask the child to let a little air out of the balloon as each mechanism is stated. Finally, discuss with the child the benefits of safely letting out one's anger when upset (Horn, 1997).

Balloon Juggling

As an ice-breaker for a beginning session of a therapy group, challenge the children to try to keep all balloons (one per person) in the air as long as possible before they touch the floor. In later sessions, the therapist can make it more challenging by adding more balloons or restrictions (e.g., use elbows or deep breaths to keep the balloons up). This activity fosters cooperation, group cohesion, and mutual enjoyment.

Message Balloon (Steer, 2003)

First, the child writes messages and/or draws pictures expressing memories of a deceased loved one. These messages are taped to a helium balloon. The child, therapist, and any support person walk to a quiet outdoor place for a release ceremony. The child is asked if he/she wishes to say anything. Then the child releases the balloon and watches its flight into the sky. An alternate technique that does not present a hazard to wildlife is to give the child a stick of incense, light it, and ask the child to watch the smoke carry a message of love up to the deceased.

Empirical Findings

A review of the literature reveals no empirical research on the balloon play technique.

Applications

Balloon play is a very enjoyable activity for children, which can elevate their mood. It can help establish rapport in individual therapy, and cohesion in child group therapy. It is also useful to teach children how to cope with anger, shyness, and bereavement.

References

Horn, T. (1997). Balloons of anger. In H. G. Kaduson & C. E. Schaefer (Eds.), *101 favorite play therapy techniques* (pp. 250–253). Northvale, NJ: Jason Aronson.

Levy, D. (1938). Release therapy in young children. *Psychiatry, 1,* 387–390.

Steer, C. (2003). The message balloon. In H. G. Kaduson & C. E. Schaefer (Eds.), *101 favorite play therapy techniques* (Vol. 3, pp. 315–316). Northvale, NJ: Jason Aronson.

Swain, H. (2010). *Make these toys: 101 clever creations using everyday items.* New York: Penguin.

11

Bop Bag Play

Holding on to anger is like grasping a hot coal with the intent of throwing it at someone else; you are the one who gets burned.
—Gautama Buddha

Introduction

The bop bag (Bobo doll) is an inflatable toy made of vinyl or plastic that stands about 4 feet tall. Introduced in the 1960s, the bop bag was advertised as a toy to help children release excess energy. The bop bag has a sand-weighted base so that it falls over and instantly lifts back up when struck. The original bop bag portrayed a clown. Modern bop bags portray a wide variety of characters including a boxer, football player, baseball player, referee, SpongeBob SquarePants, Spider-Man, and an assortment of cartoon-like animals. The "therapeutic bop bag," a 40-inch white vinyl inflatable, is blank so that children can write or draw on it with erasable markers and then strike the bag to release feelings.

Rationale

Virginia Axline (1947) described nondirective play therapy as an opportunity for children "to play out his accumulated feelings of tension, frustration, insecurity, aggression, fear, bewilderment, confusion" (p. 16). Among her list of recommended play materials, Axline included toys for expressing aggression such as toy guns and toy soldiers. Bop bags serve this function and have several therapeutic benefits, including:

• *Catharsis.* Children are often discouraged from expressing negative emotions by the adults in their lives. Bop bags help them release pent-up feelings of anger, rage, grief, and frustration (Landreth, 2002).

41

• *Self-expression.* Pent-up feelings result in anxiety, depression, and a wide variety of behavior problems in children. The action of striking a bop bag releases unexpressed, hidden, and unconscious emotions, thoughts, and conflicts. This gives therapists an understanding of the level of emotional pain, anger, or violence that children have experienced (McGuinness, 2001).

• *Relationship enhancement.* Client-centered therapists believe that providing children with the freedom to strike a bop bag and openly express negative emotions conveys a message of trust and unconditional acceptance. This shows children that they can be themselves without judgment or pressure to change and fosters a working alliance.

• *Stress relief.* Ginsburg (1993) noted that releasing negative emotions relieves tension, anxiety, and aggression, and brings about a sense of calm and relief.

Description

Ages

Three years and up.

Materials

Inflated bop bag.

Techniques

The bop bag is used in different ways depending on the orientation of the therapist. In nondirective play therapy, the bop bag is placed in the playroom where children are free to play with it whenever they wish. In directive treatment, children may be encouraged to use the bop bag to release negative feelings when they are agitated and/or in need of an outlet for angry feelings.

Regardless of the therapist's orientation, use of the bop bag requires specific limits to ensure physical safety and to prevent uncontrollable aggression and emotional flooding. Limits include that children cannot hurt themselves, the therapist, or materials in the playroom. If bop bag play becomes overstimulating or results in aggressive acting out or safety issues, the therapist needs to quickly stop the activity. If hitting the bag helps the child release negative feelings and become calmer, it has been a useful activity.

When using the bop bag in treatment, McGuinness (2001) noted the importance of reducing the connection between children's negative emotions and their aggressive behaviors. He argued that careful responses to children's expression of anger at the bop bag are vital to help children understand their underlying fear and sadness and for neutralizing their aggression. McGuinness recommended focusing on feelings and experiences conveyed by children. He offered the following case example:

> THERAPIST: You want this one to know you are angry. You would like this person to know what it feels like to be hurt. You want to tell them not to hurt you anymore.

The child is very angry but empowered: takes a sword or a gun or a baseball bat and puts a lot of energy into "hurting" the bop bag. The child spends a great deal of time beating it around the face—possible issues of identity; and the ears—perhaps indicates exposure to verbal abuse or violent arguments.

> THERAPIST: You want this one to know what it feels like to be hurt in the face, more than one time. You want this one to know what it feels like to hear things that hurt. This one needs to learn a lesson. It needs to know what it feels like to get hurt a lot.
>
> CHILD: Yeah, he needs to learn a lesson. I'm strong. (To the bop bag) How do you like it? The child continues to hit the bop bag. As the child experiences the therapist's understanding of the emotional event, the child goes deeper into his play.
>
> THERAPIST: You want this guy to know you are strong now. You have some power over this guy now. Is there anything you want to tell this guy? (pp. 325–326)

Variations

Newspaper Punch, Toss, and Free-for-All

This Theraplay technique discussed by Lindaman (2003) provides a cathartic experience for children ages 3–11 years. The technique requires six full sheets of newspaper. The therapist holds a sheet of paper taut and the child punches through the sheet. After several punches, the child and therapist crumple the sheets into balls and the child tosses them into a hoop, which the therapist makes with his/her arms. The therapist and child then toss the balls at each other to get rid of them.

Angry Kleenex Game

Introduced by Filley (2003), this technique for children of all ages requires white paper, crayons, Kleenex, a small cup of water, and tape. The therapist asks the child to think of a situation that has recently caused him/her to become frustrated or angry. The child then uses the crayons and a white sheet of paper to draw a picture, abstraction, or symbol of the person or situation. When the picture is completed, the child tapes it to a wall or door at eye level. The child then soaks a Kleenex in the cup of water, and squeezes out excess water. Standing 3–4 feet from the picture, the child hurls the Kleenex at the picture. The object of the game is to have the Kleenex be wet enough to stick to the picture. The child continues to throw wet Kleenex at the picture until he/she feels free from anger.

Tearing Pages

Show the child how to tear out pages from a phone book, crumble them, and toss into a trash can so as to rid oneself of angry feelings.

Empirical Findings

1. Bandura, Ross, and Ross (1961) found that preschoolers exposed to aggressive models were more likely to engage in aggressive behavior. In their classic Bobo doll experiment, 36 boys and 36 girls ages 3–6 years were split into three groups. Group 1 was exposed to an aggressive model, Group 2 was exposed to a nonaggressive model, and Group 3 was not exposed to a model. During the aggressive model scenario, the adult model hit, punched, threw, struck (with a mallet), and yelled at a Bobo doll. During the nonaggressive scenario, the adult played with toys and ignored the Bobo doll. Children in all groups then played freely for 20 minutes.

The results showed that children exposed to the aggressive model were more likely to imitate both physically and verbally aggressive behaviors than those who were not exposed to the aggressive model. Overall, children were more influenced by same-sex models. In addition, children who observed the nonaggressive model exhibited less mallet aggression than the control group, which had no model. Last, boys were more likely to imitate aggressive behaviors than girls.

2. Bushman, Baumeister, and Stack (1999) found that hitting a punching bag increases rather than decreases subsequent aggression. Participants in their study were divided into three groups. Group 1 read a procatharsis article, Group 2 read a neutral article, and Group 3 read an anticatharsis article. Participants then wrote an essay. To induce anger, half the participants were given negative feedback about their essay and half were given positive feedback. Subjects then chose to punch a punching bag, engage in a nonaggressive activity, or do nothing at all. People in Group 1 who received negative feedback were more likely to punch the bag than participants in Groups 1 and 2 who received negative feedback. In addition, people who received positive feedback chose to engage in nonaggressive activities.

The researchers' second study showed that engaging in cathartic behavior did not reduce anger. Participants were divided into two groups. One group struck a punching bag and the other did not. People in both groups then played a game with a fictional opponent. While playing, participants had an opportunity to punish their opponent with blasts of noise. The loudness and length of the noise were used as measures of aggression. The researchers found that people who punched the punching bag were more aggressive than people in the control group. The researchers noted that angered participants enjoyed hitting a punching bag, so at some level the activity made them feel good. They wrote that if anything, people who enjoyed hitting the punching bag more were also more aggressive toward the opponent in subsequent trials (Bushman et al., 1999, p. 375).

Applications

Bop bags are helpful for children who have inhibited the expression of angry feelings after a real-life provocation or frustration. They are also useful to help shy, inhibited individuals become more assertive, and to instill a feeling of power in children with a history of abuse, domestic violence, and injustices. The physical and emotional expression of anger stimulated by bop bags should always be accompanied with a working-through process that will enable the aggressive child to cope more adaptively with the anger-provoking situation (Bohart, 1980).

Contraindications

Striking a bop bag can cause physical arousal, enjoyment, and a sense of power in some aggressive children that can reinforce and increase the likelihood of future aggressive actions (Baumeister, Dale, & Sommer, 1998; Bushman et al., 1999). Markham (2009) argued that striking a punching bag reinforces the connection between feeling angry and acting in an aggressive manner.

Based on past research, it is important to conduct a thorough intake before allowing children to use the bop bag for venting anger. The bop bag is contraindicated for children with histories of violence or highly aggressive behavior, for those with poor impulse control, and for those who enjoy inflicting physical pain on others. In addition, it is advisable to use a blank, faceless bop bag instead of a human figure bop bag. This allows the child to release negative emotions while reducing the focus on aggression toward a person. In this regard, after a review of the literature on the catharsis theory, Bushman (2002) concluded:

> For reduction of anger and aggression, the worst possible advice to give people is to tell them to imagine their provocateur's face on a pillow or punching bag as they wallop it, yet this is precisely what many pop psychologists advise people to do. (p. 730)

References

Axline, V. M. (1947). *Play therapy: The inner dynamics of childhood*. Oxford, UK: Houghton Mifflin.

Bandura, A., Ross, D., & Ross, S. A. (1961). Transmission of aggression through imitation of aggressive models. *Journal of Abnormal and Social Psychology, 63,* 575–582.

Baumeister, R. F., Dale, K., & Sommer, K. L. (1998). Freudian defense mechanisms and empirical findings in modern social psychology: Reaction formation, projection, displacement, undoing, isolation, sublimation, and denial. *Journal of Personality, 66*(6), 1081–1124.

Bohart, A. C. (1980). Toward a cognitive theory of catharsis. *Psychotherapy: Theory, Research and Practice, 17*(2), 192–201.

Bushman, B. J. (2002). Does venting anger feed or extinguish the flame?: Catharsis, rumination, and aggressive responding. *Personality and Social Psychology Bulletin, 28*(6), 724–731.

Bushman, B., Baumeister, R., & Stack, A. (1999). Catharsis, aggression and persuasive influence: Self-fulfilling or self-defeating. *Journal of Personality and Social Psychology,* 76(3), 367–376.

Filley, D. K. (2003). Angry Kleenex game. In H. G. Kaduson & C. E. Schaefer (Eds.), *101 favorite play therapy techniques* (pp. 336–338). Lanham, MD: Jason Aronson.

Ginsberg, B. G. (1993). Catharsis. In C. E. Schaefer (Ed.), *The therapeutic powers of play* (pp. 107–141). Northvale, NJ: Jason Aronson.

Landreth, G. (2002). *Play therapy: The art of the relationship.* New York: Brunner-Routledge.

Lindaman, S. L. (2003). *101 favorite play therapy techniques* (Vol. 3). Lanham, MD: Jason Aronson.

Markham, A. (2009, September 24). You can't punch your way out of anger. *Psychology Today.* Available at *https://www.psychologytoday.com/blog/ulterior-motives/200909/you-cant-punch-your-way-out-anger.*

McGuinness, V. (2001). Therapeutic responses to the bop bag: Healing anger and aggression in children. In H. G. Kaduson & C. E. Schaefer (Eds.), *101 more favorite play therapy techniques* (pp. 323–327). Northvale, NJ: Jason Aronson.

12

Sensory Play

Introduction

Play therapy is by nature a sensory experience. Children use the senses of sight and touch when using toys and art materials; hearing when listening to music or the therapist speaking; speech when talking to the therapist; taste when food is included in treatment; and smell when scented materials such as candles, air fresheners, or scented erasers are included in the playroom.

Sensory processing involves the way in which the nervous system receives messages from the five senses and turns them into appropriate responses or behaviors. Difficulties in sensory processing occur when sensory input is not organized correctly. A. Jean Ayres, founder of the sensory integration specialty in the 1960s, compared sensory processing disorders to a neurological "traffic jam" that prevents the brain from receiving the information needed to interpret sensory signals correctly (Sensory Processing Disorder Foundation, 2015). This can manifest in challenges such as clumsiness, disruptive behaviors, anxiety, depression, academic difficulties, or problems with self-regulation.

Ayres introduced a treatment method for sensory processing difficulties that included a playful atmosphere in which sensory experiences become increasingly challenging over time. Greenspan and Wieder (2000) also developed a playful approach in which the parent uses play to join the child and gradually introduces challenges to enhance relating, communicating, and thinking. If the child is underreactive, the parent uses a lively approach. Conversely, if the child is overreactive, the parent uses a calming approach.

Rationale

Sensory play helps children engage in the world in new ways. This stimulates the senses and strengthens neural pathways, a process that contributes to the child's physical, cognitive, social, and emotional development. Sensory play has a number of therapeutic benefits, including:

• *Social skills.* Using sensory play in groups provides children with opportunities to observe how peers use materials, share their own ideas for using materials, experiment with new approaches, and enjoy the company of peers.

• *Self-confidence.* As children learn to tolerate sensory experiences, meet the challenges associated with them, and respond to them in appropriate ways, they develop confidence, pride, and self-esteem.

• *Mastery.* Because sensory play is interesting and engaging, it motivates children to overcome obstacles, which increases their interest in experimenting and ultimately improves their sensory functioning. These benefits contribute to mastery and feelings of competence.

• *Relaxation.* Sensory play helps children regulate internal discomfort related to boredom, agitation, anger, or restlessness. An activity as simple as stretching Silly Putty provides comfort and relieves stress.

• *Enjoyment and creativity.* Sensory play is process oriented. It helps children engage in the world in new ways and provides them with pleasurable experiences that promote pretend play and creativity.

Description

Ages

Two years and up.

Techniques

Sensory play can be introduced through one of the five senses or any combination of them. Tactile play includes manipulating goop, clay, sand, water, Silly Putty, beans, or beads; squeezing a stress ball; or stroking a pet or stuffed animal. Verbal play includes making animal sounds, play acting different characters, humming, or singing. Auditory play includes soothing or invigorating music; ocean, stream, or wild animal sounds found in most noise machines; playing with musical instruments; or moving a wind chime. Visual play includes drawing, painting, looking through a kaleidoscope or binoculars, blowing on a windmill, or watching the water inside a magic wand swish when turned up and down. Finally, examples of gustatory experiences include exposing children to foods with different tastes and textures.

Variations

Gloop

In this technique introduced by Cabe (1997) the therapist works with the child to make play clay or personal Silly Putty, which Cabe called "gloop." Play clay is a mixture of flour, salt, water, and vegetable oil. Food coloring and flavoring can also be added if the child wishes. Gloop, which is much more fluid, is a mixture of Elmer's Glue, water, and 20 Mule Team Borax laundry powder. One or both mediums are used to make characters and objects that the child may choose to take home at the end of the session.

Shaving Cream

In this technique (Greenberg, 2003), the therapist places a can of shaving cream with other materials such as paints, clay, and crayons, and informs children that they can choose whatever materials they would like to play with. Children can spray shaving cream on a table, smear it, dig into it, and make shapes and objects with it. They can spread it onto their hands and arms and pretend that they are shaving. Some children enjoy mixing shaving cream with water in a dishpan and beating it with an eggbeater to make bubbles. In addition to enjoying the feel and malleability of shaving cream, many children take pleasure in its lingering scent.

Lotion Game

This Theraplay technique (Rieff, 2003) requires lotion and cotton balls. The session begins with the therapist counting and nurturing the child's "boo-boos" with lotion. After doing so, the therapist may stick a cotton ball with lotion on his/her own nose and both the child and therapist try blowing it off. After several rounds, the therapist throws sticky, lotion-covered cotton balls at the wall and encourages the child to do the same. These activities help the child learn to regulate sensory input. The technique may be adapted based on the needs and tolerance of the child. For some children, just counting boo-boos may be appropriate. Others may tolerate more sensory experiences.

Empirical Findings

Gourley, Wind, Henninger, and Chinitz (2013) examined the relationship among sensory processing difficulties, parental stress, and behavioral problems in a sample of urban children ages 2–5 years. The sample consisted of 59 children who had been identified with developmental and behavioral difficulties. Parents completed the Child Behavior Checklist, the Parental Stress Inventory—Short Form, and the Short Sensory Profile. The children showed a high prevalence (55.9%) of sensory processing difficulties, which were correlated with behavioral difficulties and parental stress levels. The results indicated that as difficulties with sensory processing increase, behavioral difficulties and parental stress also increase.

Applications

Sensory play helps children tolerate sensory experiences in a fun, gradual way, which empowers them to overcome processing difficulties. It is an ideal medium for children with sensory integration difficulties and problems with self-regulation. In addition, sensory play can be used to reduce arousal in children with histories of abuse, neglect, and trauma. Children with ADHD, anxiety disorders, spectrum disorders, and depression benefit from the soothing qualities of sensory play. Also, playing with gooey substances such as Play Dough and wet sand may lessen a child's urge to play with bodily wastes, or hold back "icky" feces, which can result in encopresis.

References

Cabe, N. (1997). Gloop: Treating sensory deprivation. In H. G. Kaduson & C. E. Schaefer (Eds.), *101 favorite play therapy techniques* (pp. 83–86). Northvale, NJ: Jason Aronson.

Gourley, L., Wind, C., Henninger, E. M., & Chinitz, S. (2013) Sensory processing difficulties, behavior problems, and parental stress in a clinical population of young children. *Journal of Child and Family Studies, 22*(7), 912–921.

Greenburg, C. H. (2003). Shaving cream. In H. G. Kaduson & C. E. Schaefer (Eds.), *101 favorite play therapy techniques* (Vol. 3, pp. 282–285). Northvale, NJ: Jason Aronson.

Greenspan S. I., & Weider, S. (2000). Developmentally appropriate interventions and practices. *Clinical Practice Guidelines* (pp. 265–266). Bethesda, MD: ICDL Press.

Rieff, M. L. (2003). The lotion game: A theraplay technique. In H. G. Kaduson & C. E. Schaefer (Eds.), *101 favorite play therapy techniques* (Vol. 3, pp. 143–144). Northvale, NJ: Jason Aronson.

Sensory Processing Disorder Foundation. (2015). About SPD. Retrieved from *http://spdfoundation.net/about-sensory-processing-disorder.html*.

Part Two

METAPHORS AND STORYTELLING TECHNIQUES

13

Concrete Play Metaphors

Introduction

Metaphors have been used since biblical times to open the mind to new ways of thinking and acting. While metaphors have long been part of traditional healing methods, clinicians of different orientations are rediscovering their use in play therapy. A metaphor is a thought process wherein one thing is expressed in terms of another. A prop is a concrete object, such as a toy, that the therapist transforms into a metaphoric object that is relevant therapeutically. Props can transform abstract concepts into concrete representations that can be seen, touched, and played with. This makes them more easily understood by young children who think primarily in images rather than abstract verbalizations (Walawander, 2007).

Rationale

There are two main therapeutic functions of metaphors with children, namely:

- *Self-expression.* Props can provide the natural language for a child to express concerns, desires, and emotions that cannot be easily or fully explained in words.
- *New learning.* Concrete metaphors can help children understand difficult, abstract concepts by connecting them with familiar images from ordinary life experiences. Interesting props can also heighten a child's interest in learning.

Description

Ages

Four to 10 years.

Techniques

Fuse

In this technique developed by Schimmel and Jacobs (2011), the therapist shows a child who angers easily two pieces of string, one an inch long and the other a foot long. The therapist explains that a person with this very short fuse (string) tends to get angry and explode (yell, scream, fight, get into trouble) more quickly than someone with a longer fuse. The therapist then points out that with a longer fuse one has time to think and react better to the situation than just blowing up. The therapist then asks the child if he/she would like to be taught how to get a longer fuse.

Metaphorical Family

First, provide the child with a diverse selection of 25–30 miniature toys, including figurines with both positive and negative association, such as tame and wild animals, insects, and fantasy characters (witches, dragons, fairies, and royalty family). Next, ask the child to select a miniature that best represents each of his/her family members, including a self-figure—for example, a child might choose a bug to represent his mother ("She's always bugging me"), a scorpion to represent his father ("He hits me and hurts me"), and a Santa Claus to represent his grandfather ("He likes to buy me things"). Alternately, each member of a family can be asked to choose a miniature to represent each of the other family members.

Externalizing Feelings

Ask the child to select a miniature toy animal to reflect each of his/her moods (e.g., a ferocious tiger for anger, a vulnerable mouse for fear). Then brainstorm with the child ways to overcome the maladaptive behaviors associated with these feeling figures.

My Shadow

Ask the child to pick a miniature figure or object that represents his/her "dark side."

Balloon Pop

A balloon can be inflated until it pops to represent feelings of anger that can build up inside yourself until you explode with aggressive behaviors (see Chapter 10, "Balloon Play").

Empirical Findings

The concrete play metaphors technique is in need of empirical research.

Applications

Concrete metaphors are a useful way for therapists to transform abstract concepts into tangible ideas and concrete representations that make them more easily understood by children. This enables therapists to teach children about issues in a way that is meaningful and age appropriate. Metaphors are also a useful way to help children express issues and concerns. They can be used with children with a wide variety of presenting problems.

References

Schimmel, C., & Jacobs, E. (2011). Ten creative counseling techniques for helping clients deal with anger. Retrieved from *http://counselingoutfitters.com/vists/vista11/article_53.pdf.*
Walawander, C. (2007). *The therapeutic use of props.* Ann Arbor, MI: Proquest.

14

Turtle Technique

Introduction

The turtle technique was initially created to teach adults to control their anger but child clinicians and educators have adapted it for similar use with preschool- and school-age children (Greenberg, Kusche, Cook, & Quamma, 1995; Robin, Schneider, & Dolnick, 1976; Schneider, 1974; Webster-Stratton & Hammond, 1997). The technique is a method for helping children to calm themselves and control disruptive behaviors. Developed by Schneider and Robin (1974), the turtle technique combines anger and impulse control strategies that help children identify anger, learn to control it, and find ways to deal with upsetting situations. This is done by using the metaphor of a turtle that withdraws into its shell when it feels threatened. Children are taught to withdraw into their imaginary shell when they feel overwhelmed by uncontrollable emotions or upsetting events that make them want to lash out.

Rationale

Studies have shown that children who exhibit aggressive behaviors at an early age are at greater risk for developing antisocial behaviors that persist into adulthood (Kazdin, 1987; Walker et al., 1996). Many children with conduct problems lack the requisite skills to control their angry outburst to provocations, disappointments, and frustrations. Just telling such children to "calm down" is not likely to change their feelings or behavior. Teaching an effective problem-solving skill through a playful metaphor of a turtle can be a successful alternative.

The turtle technique brings about internal changes in children as well as external effects on the environment. The therapeutic benefits of the technique include:

• *Self-expression.* The turtle technique helps children learn to express feelings in healthy ways. Schneider and Robin (1974) wrote:

> When a child impulsively lashes out at his environment, he may be expressing raw emotion, but the consequences of his display of feeling may be negative for him and for others. Through the Turtle Technique, we teach the child to channel his expression of emotions in appropriate ways: instead of lashing out, the child learns to define his needs (i.e., for affection, attention, easier work, a pencil, etc.) and to seek the satisfaction of these needs with a pro-social expression of emotion. In essence, we try to teach the distinction between assertion and aggression. (p. 9)

• *Prosocial behavior.* When children do the turtle technique instead of reacting to a peer's problematic behaviors, the disruptive child does not receive the attention he/she previously had for inappropriate behavior.

• *Metaphorical teaching.* Withdrawing into a shell and relaxing gives children an alternative method for dealing with frustrations and coping with strong emotions. In addition, the problem-solving aspect of this technique teaches children how to deal with frustrations and get needs met in healthy ways.

• *Creative thinking.* The turtle technique promotes the idea of coming up with innovative solutions to problems. This promotes flexibility in thoughts and actions.

• *Self-esteem.* The ability to control internal feelings boosts children's self-esteem because it provides a sense of mastery and competence.

Description

Ages

The turtle technique works well with individual and groups of children, ages 4–8 years, in therapy and classroom settings (Schneider & Robin, 1974).

Materials

Turtle puppet or paper-plate model of a turtle.

Techniques

Begin by explaining that the turtle model you are holding has learned a special trick for calming down when upset. First, he recognizes that he is feeling angry. Next, he thinks to himself "STOP!" He then goes into his shell, pulls his arms and legs tightly to his body, closes his eyes, lowers his head, takes three deep breaths, and thinks calming thoughts such as "I can be calm and think of good solutions." Finally, the turtle comes out of his shell when calm and thinks of solutions to the problem. The child can practice this four-step process with the turtle puppet or a paper-plate turtle with a moveable head and arms that go into their shell. Pictures of the turtle technique available on the Internet can be used to remind a child of the steps for calming down. The original "Turtle Manual" by Schneider and Robin (1974) is also available on the Internet from Google.

The turtle technique has been used to teach individual and groups of children a skill that combines imagery, problem solving, and relaxation to help them solve problems without acting aggressively. To promote generalization, the therapist can share the technique with teachers and parents. Once the turtle technique is learned, a visual signal to prompt children to use the technique when agitated is for an adult to raise a hand and clench it—symbolizing a turtle going into its shell.

Empirical Findings

1. Heffner, Greco, and Eifert (2003) found that preschoolers favored receiving metaphorical relaxation instructions ("Pretend you are a turtle going into its shell") over literal relaxation instruction ("Squeeze your shoulders up to your ears").

2. Robin and colleagues (1976) investigated the use of the turtle technique to help emotionally disturbed children improve their self-control of aggression. The results revealed a significant decrease in aggressive behavior in the classroom.

3. Bethell, Newacheck, Hawes, and Halfon (2014) found that children ages 6–17 years with the ability to stay calm and in control when faced with challenges were better able to ameliorate the negative impact of stressful life events.

Applications

The turtle technique can foster resilience in children who experienced trauma. It also helps children with conduct problems learn adaptive problem-solving skills and thus inhibits their impulsive, aggressive response to provocations, such as teasing.

References

Bethell, C., Newacheck, P., Hawes, E., & Halfon, N. (2014). Adverse childhood experiences: Assessing the impact on health and school engagement and the mitigating role of resiliency. *Health Affairs, 33*(12), 2106–2115.

Greenberg, M. T., Kusche, C., Cook, E., & Quamma, J. (1995). Promoting emotional competence in school-aged children: The effects of the PATHS curriculum. *Development and Psychopathology, 7*, 127–136.

Heffner, M., Greco, L., & Eifert, G. (2003). Pretend you are a turtle: Children's responses to metaphorical versus literal relaxation instructions. *Child and Family Behavior Therapy, 25*(1), 19–33.

Kazdin, A. E. (1987). Treatment of antisocial behavior in children. *Psychological Bulletin*, *102*(27), 187–203.

Robin, A., Schneider, M., & Dolnick, M. (1976). The turtle technique: An extended case study of self-control in the classroom. *Psychology in the Schools*, *13*, 449–453.

Schneider, M. (1974). Turtle technique in the classroom. *Teaching Exceptional Children*, *7*(1), 22–24.

Schneider, M., & Robin, A. (1974). Turtle manual. Retrieved from *http://files.eric.ed.gov/fulltext/ED128680.pdf.*

Walker, H., Horner, R., Sugai, G., Bullis, M., Sprague, J., Brisker, D., et al. (1996). Integrated approaches to preventing antisocial behavior problems among school-age children and youth. *Journal of Emotional and Behavior Disorders*, *4*(4), 194–209.

Webster-Stratton, C., & Hammond, M. (1997). Treating children with early-onset conduct problems: A comparison of child and parent training interventions. *Journal of Consulting and Clinical Psychology*, *65*(1), 93–109.

15

Emotion Thermometer

Introduction

Therapists have used client self-assessment scales to obtain information for setting treatment goals and evaluating progress for several decades—for example, Wolpe (1969) developed the Subjective Units of Distress Scale (SUDS) for measuring the subjective intensity of psychological distress experienced by a client. Moreover, narrative therapists frequently use the scaling technique to help clients rate the severity of their disturbance on a scale of 0 to 10 (Guterman, 2006).

Many child therapists have employed the visual metaphor of a thermometer to enable children to rate the intensity of their emotions. A thermometer is familiar to children as an instrument with a graduated glass tube and bulb containing an indicator that rises and falls when one's internal temperature changes. Similarly, an emotion thermometer is a visual tool used to help children rate the intensity of their internal feelings. It has been used for over 40 years as a visual analogue scale to assess clients' self-reported mood states (Ahearn, 1997).

The emotion thermometer provides a measure of the intensity of a feeling on a continuum from low to high. It is often marked with lines or gradations that are numbered or labeled with words or pictures depicting the strength of the emotion. The child is often asked to color in the appropriate level on the thermometer to depict the intensity of his/her internal feeling, such as anger, fear, or happiness.

Rationale

Children tend to think in black and white extremes and have difficulty understanding the fact that feelings exist on a continuum. Emotion thermometers provide an age-appropriate way for children to learn about the subtleties and gradations of feelings and behaviors. Their therapeutic benefits include:

- *Self-expression.* Pictures and other visual metaphors enable children to express the intensity of feeling states they may not have words to describe (Bries-meister, 2001).

- *Self-awareness.* Emotion thermometers give children a tool for understanding their feelings and the people, situations, and circumstances that make feelings escalate and decrease.

- *Positive emotion.* Emotion thermometers are engaging and fun to color and create. They can be adapted to the specific needs and personalities of children to make them humorous and/or relatable.

Description

Ages

Five years and up.

Materials

Free emotion thermometer templates are available on the Internet.

Techniques

Most children are familiar with thermometers and understand that parents use them when they are sick. The therapist can introduce the idea of an emotion thermometer by showing the child a picture of one. Alternately, the therapist can draw an individualized emotion thermometer to address the child's specific emotional and developmental needs prior to the session or by making one with the child. Freeman and Garcia (2008) offer the following dialogue to introduce the feelings thermometer:

> A feeling thermometer is just like other thermometers only it measures feelings instead of temperature. Knowing how you feel or how much you feel something will help us work together in this treatment. Here is a picture of a feeling thermometer. At the top of the picture next to the frowning face is the number 10. If you rated something with a frowning face and a number 10 that would mean that you felt really bad or anxious about the situation you were rating. At the bottom of the picture is a smiling face and the number 0. If you rated something with a smiling face and a 0 that would mean that you didn't feel anxious or bad about the situation you were rating. Imagine that in the middle is a picture of neither a smile nor a frown and the number 5. What should we call this kind of face? (If the child doesn't offer an option, suggest calling it medium face.) This means that you feel some anxiety or bad feelings about the situation you are rating. Can you give me some examples of things that you would rate with a smiley face? A medium face? And a frowning face? (p. 65)

Variations

Fluster-ometer

Rubin (2003) designed this technique for children of all ages. The fluster-ometer is a dial made with cardboard that includes a needle or fluster arrow, held in place with a pushpin so it can move from left to right. The dial has three zones: green (cruising zone), yellow (fluster zone), and red (brain block). Bubble spaces are included for each zone with messages that children tell themselves. Examples for the green zone include "I know this" and "This is easy." Examples for the yellow zone include "I should know this" and "Why can't I get it?" Examples for the red zone include "I am stupid" and "I'll never know this." The therapist and child adapt these messages to the child's level of frustration in meeting challenging tasks at school or in play situations. Thus, when the child becomes flustered in performing tasks in the playroom, such as game play, the child and therapist position the dial to whatever zone the child is or was experiencing. The dial is then repositioned after relaxation techniques are used. Rubin notes that "monitoring the downward movement of the dial while using anxiety reducing techniques is the immediate goal, while implementing them outside of the therapy room is the long-term challenge" (p. 292).

Stressometer

The authors of Golden Path Games (2014) designed this printable assessment tool for clients ages 7 years through adulthood. The stressometer provides individuals with a visual tool to assess the impact of stress in their lives and includes three parts: a thought bubble used to identify sources of stress, a feeling chart used to explore emotional responses to specific stressors, and a stress thermometer used to determine how well the individual is coping with that stressor. The technique starts with a discussion about healthy and unhealthy stress. The child uses the thought bubble to identify healthy and unhealthy stressors in his/her life and chooses one specific stressor to discuss. Emotions associated with that stressor are reviewed and the child colors the thermometer to reflect how much stress he/she is experiencing with it. A conversation about whether the child's stress is healthy or unhealthy follows, with a focus on helpful coping skills.

Emotional Barometer

Elliot (2002) developed the emotional barometer as a graphic aid designed to help children ages 5–12 years discuss feelings and moods. The barometer has two ends that range from 0 (*Life is the pits*), to 10 (*Life is great*). At the start of each session, children are asked to draw a line on the barometer to show how things are going for them. Sometimes children use different colors and relate them to feelings about home, school, and friendships. Helping children discuss concerns in this way makes them concrete and manageable.

The Feeling and Doing Thermometer

In this technique developed by Briesmeister (2001), a large thermometer is drawn on an art board or piece of cardboard with gradations from 1 to 5 drawn on the outside of it. The bottom section is cut out and a smaller strip of red paper is placed behind the cut-out section. An identical blue strip is also made. Children are instructed to measure the level of their feeling states by sliding the red strip to the matching intensity. The blue strip is used to measure the intensity of their behavioral states. This technique helps children regulate feelings and behaviors. It can be adapted for young children by using puppets to teach them about feelings.

How Many Degrees?

Macklem (2010) introduced this as a small-group activity for children ages 8 years and up. The objective of the activity is to help children connect a number to the intensity of an emotion word. First, a feeling thermometer with numbers on a continuum from 1 to 6 is presented and an emotion is stated, such as anger. The children take turns rolling the die and think of a word that describes the intensity of that emotion based on the number shown on the die—for example, if the die shows a 6 and the emotion being discussed is anger, the word he/she comes up with must convey intense anger (e.g., *furious*).

Alternate Visual Metaphors

Freeman and Garcia (2008) describe a number of visual metaphors (apart from a thermometer) to help children rate the level of their feelings—for example, the metaphor of carrying heavy bricks can be used by a child to draw the number of bricks that reflect the amount of burden he/she is currently experiencing in a particular situation. Similarly, a child can use the metaphor of butterflies in the tummy to draw the number of butterflies that reflect his/her present level of anxiety.

Empirical Findings

1. Wyman and colleagues (2010) found that children taught to monitor and control anger and other emotions showed improved classroom behavior and had significantly fewer discipline problems and suspensions. Two hundred and twenty-six kindergarten to third-grade children identified with elevated behavioral and social classroom problems participated in the program. Mentors taught children in the study group about feelings and used feelings thermometers to teach self-control and regulation of emotions. Children learned to use "mental muscles" to monitor feelings and to stop feelings from entering the part of the thermometer labeled the *hot zone*. They also learned to use breathing exercises and guided imagery to maintain control and regain equilibrium. Children who received training showed

improved classroom behaviors and fewer disciplinary incidents. They also showed less aggressive or disruptive behaviors and improved on-task learning behaviors. Socially, they were less withdrawn and more assertive.

2. A study by Beck, Tan, Lum, Lim, and Krishna (2014) found that emotion thermometers are valid and reliable instruments for assessing distress, anxiety, and depression in cancer patients.

Applications

Emotion thermometers provide a way for children to identify, monitor, and regulate feelings, thoughts, and behaviors. This makes them an extremely valuable tool for children with a wide range of presenting difficulties. Emotion thermometers can be used to help children recognize and gauge the extent of their internal states related to fear, anxiety, depression, anger, perfectionism, and social inhibition. They also provide a way for the therapist to monitor changes in these emotions over time. The emotion thermometer technique can be applied in individual, group, and family therapy as well as classroom settings.

References

Ahearn, E. P. (1997). The use of visual analog scales in mood disorders: A critical review. *Journal of Psychiatric Research, 5,* 569–579.

Beck, K. R., Tan, S., Lum, S., Lim, L., & Krishna, L. (2014). Validation of the emotion thermometers and hospital anxiety and depression scales in Singapore: Screening cancer patients for distress, anxiety and depression. *Asia-Pacific Journal of Clinical Oncology.* Retrieved from *http://onlinelibrary.wiley.com/doi/10.1111/ajco.12180/abstract.*

Briesmeister, J. M. (2001). The "feeling" and "doing" thermometer: A technique for self-monitoring. In H. G. Kaduson & C. E. Schaefer (Eds.), *101 more favorite play therapy techniques* (pp. 98–102). Northvale, NJ: Jason Aronson.

Elliott, S. (2002). The emotional barometer. In C. E. Schaefer & D. M. Cangelosi (Eds.), *Play therapy techniques* (2nd ed.). Northvale, NJ: Jason Aronson.

Freeman, J. B., & Garcia, A. M. (2008). *Family based treatment for young children with OCD.* New York: Oxford University Press.

Golden Path Games. (2014). Stressometer. Retrieved from *www.playtherapyworks.com/uploads/2/3/7/7/2377039/stressometer5_2014.10.pdf.*

Guterman, J. T. (2006). *Mastering the art of solution-focused counseling.* Alexandria, VA: American Counseling Association.

Macklem, G. L. (2010). *Evidence-based school mental health services: Affect education, emotion regulation training and cognitive behavioral therapy.* New York: Springer.

Rubin, L. (2003). The Fluster-ometer. In H. G. Kaduson & C. E. Schaefer (Eds.), *101 favorite play therapy techniques* (Vol. 3, pp. 290–293). Lanham, MD: Jason Aronson.

Wolpe, J. (1969). *The practice of behavior therapy.* New York: Pergamon Press.

Wyman, P. A., Cross, W., Brown, C. H., Yu, Q., Tu, X., & Eberly, S. (2010). Intervention to strengthen emotional self-regulation in children with emerging mental health problems: Proximal impact on school behavior. *Journal of Abnormal Child Psychology, 38*(5), 707–720.

16

Storytelling

> After nourishment, shelter and companionship, stories are the thing
> we need most in the world.
>
> —PHILIP PULLMAN

Introduction

A story is a narrative—a telling about a certain event or events that happened to certain people at a specific time and place. Storytelling is as ancient as language itself and reflects the human need to communicate experiences to other human beings (Pellowski, 1977). Everything that happens to us in life is filed at the back of our minds in containers called "stories" (Barton, 1987). The storytelling technique with children has been an important clinical intervention since the first two decades of the 20th century. It includes a family of techniques, which includes child storytelling, mutual storytelling, and therapist storytelling.

CHILD STORYTELLING

Rationale

Stories allow children to express their thoughts and feelings and thus gain a deeper understanding of themselves.

Description

Ages

Three to 12 years.

Through storytelling, children develop a personal voice, expressing their unique way of thinking and feeling about themselves. Like other forms of fantasy, children's stories reflect their conscious and unconscious experiences, emotions, and desires. Three-year-olds may attempt to tell a story using phrases and short sentences, but they can only sustain it with much questioning and prompting from an adult. By the age of 4 years, children pick up on conventional storytelling devices, such as "Once upon a time" and "The end" and become more fluent in telling a tale. This age is the imaginative peak for children's stories. The action is seldom bound by the restraints of reality. While the plots of young children often involve eating, sleeping, and the appearance of a kindly figure, violence is the predominant theme. Typically, they tell stories about monsters, death, killing, and crashing. The stories are their way of dealing with fears and feelings of aggression. By age 3 years, telling a story about oneself or others becomes an important way for children to make sense of the world. Around 8 years of age children's thinking has developed enough for them to apply general principles to concrete situations—that is, state the lesson of their story, and tell stories with a beginning, middle, and an end. The beginning introduces the characters and setting, the middle describes the problem, and the end presents the resolution.

Techniques

Children are natural storytellers and enjoy telling their own stories. However, young children often need help in expressing their stories, in the form of starters, prompts, and inquiries.

- *Starters.* One way to ensure that a child tells an original story is to suggest that the story begin with the phrase "Once upon a time," or "Once upon a time, a long, long time ago, in a land far away." Such openers immediately create the expectation by both storyteller and listener that the story will be about the land of make-believe (Mutchnick & Handler, 2002).

- *Prompts.* As the child tells a story, he/she may need to be prompted to continue the story. The most common, open-ended prompt is "Then what happened?" The tone of the therapist's question should convey interest and genuine curiosity so that the storytelling experience remains fun for the child. Most children bring their stories to a natural conclusion. Some include a closing statement, such as "The end" or "That's all."

- *Inquiries.* It is helpful for the therapist to engage in a poststory dialogue in which he/she asks questions to clarify ambiguous elements of the child's story and establishes parallels between the story and issues in the child's life.

Variations

Object-Based Stories

Preschoolers (ages 3–5 years) enjoy using props to tell stories—for example, for a child who is an outcast at school, his therapist might provide him with a group of elephant toy miniatures, including one purple elephant, and ask him to tell a story using the miniatures. Another adaptation is to use Richard Gardner's "Pick-and-Tell Game" and ask a child to pick a miniature toy object from a bag and tell a story about it. Alternately, a therapist may collect small toys and objects and put them in a bag so the child can reach in and remove one to tell a story about. The objective of this "bag of objects" technique is to facilitate young children's expression of their innermost feelings and concerns.

"Story stems" or doll play completions are another object-based variation. They are particularly useful for uncovering children's perceptions of family relationships (Buchsbaum & Emde, 1992; Cassidy, 1988; Warren, Oppenheim, & Emde, 1996). The therapist or interviewer uses miniature doll house dolls and furniture to present the child with a number of potentially challenging home situations (e.g., the child doll spills milk while the doll family is dining together). The child is asked to tell and show what happens next.

The following are additional story stems from the MacArthur Story Stem Battery (Warren et al., 1996):

- *Scary dog.* In a park, the child kicks a ball away from the family. Suddenly, a scary dog appears and barks loudly.
- *Monsters in the dark.* It's nighttime and the child is alone. Suddenly the lights go out and the child thinks he/she hears a monster.
- *Canceled visit.* The child has been looking forward to visiting with a friend but Mom tells the child that he/she can't go.
- *Fight with friends.* While the child is playing with his/her ball, the child's friend grabs it, hurting the child's hand.

Numerous research findings on the story stem technique have found that this play enactment provides a reliable and valid window into the family relations of children ages 3–8 years (Salmon, 2006).

Picture-Based Stories

Ask the child to tell a story about evocative pictures you present, such as from magazines, or from assessment instruments such as the Children's Apperception Test (CAT) or the Thematic Apperception Test (TAT; Bellak, 1954).

Alternating Line Stories

One child starts the story and each person in the group adds a line to it. This group storytelling technique stimulates attention, working memory, and self-control in children.

MUTUAL STORYTELLING

The mutual storytelling technique developed by child psychiatrist Richard Gardner (1971) is a well-known technique involving the telling of stories by both the child and the therapist. Mutual storytelling does not require specific talent for storytelling or any highly specialized training. All that is needed is a willingness to be creative and have some fun in the process.

Description

Ages

Eight to 14 years.

Techniques

Gardner (1983) recommended initiating the technique as follows:

> I begin by asking the child if he or she would like to be a guest of honor on a make-believe television program on which stories are told. If the child agrees—and few decline the honor—the tape recorder is turned on and I begin: "Good morning boys and girls, ladies and gentlemen. I'm happy to welcome you once again to Dr. Gardner's 'Make-Up-a-Story Television Program.' On this program, we invite children to see how good they are at making up stories. It's against the rules to tell any stories about anything that really happened to you or anyone you know. The story cannot be about anything you've seen on television, heard on the radio, or read in books. Naturally, the more adventure or excitement the story has, the more fun it will be to watch on television afterward. After you finish your story, you tell us the moral or lesson of your story. And everyone knows that every good story has a lesson or moral." (pp. 356–357)

Then, Gardner makes up a story and tells the lesson or moral of his story.

After the child's story, Gardner tells a story of his own using the same characters, story line, and setting as in the child's story. His goal is to introduce more adaptive resolutions to the problems and conflicts that have been expressed in the child's story. Gardner believed that insights provided in story form bypass the conscious mind and are received directly by the child's unconscious mind. He also maintained that when a therapist uses stories to speak in a child's own language, there is a greater likelihood that the message will be heard and internalized by the child.

For example, a 6-year-old boy told a story of a mama bear and little baby bear who were hungry so they went into the woods looking for food. They found a beehive full of honey and no bees around. The mama bear knocked the hive down from the tree and began licking the honey. She was so hungry that she kept licking and licking and forgot about baby bear. Finally, when the honey was all gone she gave the hive to baby bear who just sat down and cried. Moral: In this family everyone looks out for themselves.

The therapist retold the first part of the story and then said, "Mama bear fell asleep after eating the honey. Really hungry now, baby bear went across the forest to Aunt Bertha's house where she fed him milk and honey. Moral: If a child keeps looking, he'll find an adult to care for him."

Variation

Alternating Story Lines

The therapist starts the story or provides the setting and then the therapist and child take turns adding a story line. Continue until either one wants to end the story.

THERAPIST STORYTELLING

From ancient times, adults have used storytelling (e.g., myths, legends, fables) as powerful teaching and healing tools. Stories tell us how to live, how to cope with difficult situations, and how to resolve problems. Human beings are hardwired to share their experiences with others, and there is a storyteller in every adult waiting to be awakened. Stories are potent because children pay attention to and absorb the metaphorical insights embedded in the stories, whereas they tend to tune out if they receive the same information while being lectured to by an adult (Brandell, 2000). From characters in stories, children can gain insights that help them solve their own problems.

Creating a story for a child is more beneficial than reading a storybook because personalized stories capture each child's unique personality and therapeutic needs. Knowledge of a child's specific interests and situation helps the therapist develop a tailor-made story that makes the child feel special, understood, and nurtured.

Rationale

Davis (1989, p. 18) noted: "Therapeutic stories appear to be particularly effective because they are nonthreatening, bypass natural resistance to change, model flexibility, make a presented idea more memorable, and mobilize the problem-solving and healing resources of the unconscious."

Description

Ages

Three to 12 years.

Techniques

The first step in creating a story for a child is to select a therapeutic metaphor and/or prop that is relevant to the child's problem or situation—for example, a grieving child might be told a story about a rabbit whose sibling or parent has died. A child of divorce might be told a story of a litter of puppies that lost their mother. Metaphors and/or props help extend and enrich a story and are often best found from the child or situation (e.g., the child's favorite animal, toy, superhero, or cartoon character). The story line is as important an ingredient as the positive resolution, since the story line helps build the story's tension, involving several turnings and tasks in the process.

Stories need to be age appropriate and teach indirectly, not by preaching. For instance, a story about a boy whose mom gives him a stern look and a talking to after he hurt his friend—is a lecture, not a story. Bruno Bettelheim in his book *The Uses of Enchantment* (1976) emphasized that it is unnecessary to interpret stories for children; rather, they should be allowed to come to their own conclusion.

When first telling stories, adults feel uncomfortable and make mistakes. However, with practice they gradually develop this skill and come to enjoy it. A practical guide to storytelling, entitled *Tell a Story—Solve a Problem* was developed by William Cook and is available as a free e-book download from his website (*www. drbillcook.com*).

For example, Mills, Crowley, and O'Ryan (1986) described a case of an 8-year-old girl who was told the story "The Monsters and the Cupcake." The girl was experiencing a fear of monsters in her bedroom that resulted in sleeplessness. The story recounted how monsters were really make-believe disguises by unhappy children who had no friends. These friendless children dressed up like monsters to gain lots of attention in order to get the other children to notice and like them, but instead, they only succeeded in scaring the other children away. The child was then asked to describe how the monster might feel from her observation of the movie *E.T.* (Spielberg, 1982) and how the boy Elliot had given E.T. a gift so as to initiate friendship. The child was asked to go home and do the same for her monsters; thus the cupcake was chosen. Over the course of several weeks of verbal reminders and multiple cupcakes, the child was able to sleep well.

Variation

Creative Characters

In the "creative characters" technique (Brooks, 1993), the therapist selects the major emotional issues confronting the child and then develops characters (quite often animals) and involves these characters in situations reflecting the core issues in therapy. These characters and the experiences they face are typically elaborated upon by the child and therapist over a number of months.

Empirical Findings

The various types of storytelling techniques with children are in need of empirical research.

Applications

Storytelling in its various forms is a very adaptable technique that can be used across a wide variety of childhood problems, including fears, anxieties, depression, low self-esteem, aggression, and trauma. It is particularly appropriate with children experiencing illness, death, divorce, bullying, or other life transitions or crises.

Contraindications

Certain children with developmental disabilities may not possess the minimal cognitive resources required for even the most elementary story.

References

Barton, B. (1987). *Tell me another.* Toronto: Nelson Thornes.

Bellak, L. (1954). *The TAT and CAT in clinical use.* New York: Grune & Stratton.

Bettleheim, B. (1976). *The uses of enchantment.* New York: Knoff.

Brandell, J. (2000). *Of mice and metaphor: Therapeutic storytelling with children.* New York: Basic Books.

Brooks, R. (1993). Creative characters. In C. E. Schaefer & D. Cangelosi (Eds.), *Play therapy techniques* (pp. 211–224). Lanham, MD: Jason Aronson.

Buchsbaum, H., Toth, S., & Emde, R. (1992). The use of narrative story stem technique with maltreated children. *Developmental Psychopathology, 4,* 603–625.

Cassidy, J. (1988). Child–mother attachment and the self in six-year-olds. *Child Development, 59,* 121–134.

Davis, N. (1989). The use of therapeutic stories in the treatment of abused children. *Journal of Strategic and Systemic Therapies, 8*(4), 18–23.

Gardner, R. (1971). *Therapeutic communication with children: The mutual storytelling technique.* New York: Jason Aronson.

Gardner, R. (1983). Mutual storytelling technique. In C. Schaefer & K. O'Connor (Eds.), *Handbook of play therapy.* New York: Wiley.

Miles, J., Crowley, R., & O'Ryan, M. (1986). *Therapeutic metaphors for children and the child within.* New York: Brunner/Mazel.

Mutchnick, M., & Handler, L. (2002). Once upon a time . . . , therapeutic interactive stories. *Humanist Psychologist, 30,* 75–84.

Pellowski, A. (1977). *The world of storytelling.* New York: Bowler.

Salmon, K. (2006). Toys in clinical interviews with children: Review and implications for practice. *Clinical Psychologist, 10*(20), 54–59.

Spielberg, S. (Director). (1982). *E.T.: The extra-terrestrial* [Motion picture]. United States: Universal City Studios.

Warren, S., Oppenheim, D., & Emde, R. (1996). Can emotions and themes in children's play predict behavioral problems? *Journal of the American Academy of Child and Adolescent Psychiatry, 35*(10), 1331–1337.

17

Externalization Play

Introduction

Externalization means to put something outside its original borders, especially to put a human function outside the human body. In Freudian psychology, externalization is an unconscious defense mechanism, whereby an individual "projects" his/her own internal characteristics onto the outside world, particularly onto other people. Thus, a client who is argumentative might instead perceive others as argumentative and him/herself as blameless. Like other defense mechanisms, projection is a protection against anxiety and is, therefore, part of a normal functioning mind.

Winnicott (1971) was one of the first therapists to point out that pretend play allows children to project inner psychological problems onto play objects and thus externalize them. The externalized self-object is then perceived as "other" so that the player can interact with it and gain control over it in imaginative play. This enables players to change and heal themselves.

Rationale

In the externalization technique, clients are helped to use the externalization process in a conscious, deliberate way. The primary goal of this narrative therapy technique (White & Epston, 1990) is to help children externalize their problems and thereby separate the individual from his/her problems. In fact, the maxim is "The problem is the problem, the person is not the problem." When a child believes the problem is part of his/her personality, it leads to feelings of guilt and embarrassment. Also, it is difficult to make changes and to call on inner resources to make those changes. Moving the focus of the problem outside the child relieves the pressure of blame and guilt and frees the therapist and client to focus on ways to overcome the problem.

72

Description

Ages

Four years and up.

Techniques

The therapist and child work together to create a character depicting the child's problem. A drawing, painting, or collage of the presenting problem is a natural way of separating the person from the problem because through art the problem becomes something visible. A toy can also be used as a metaphoric prop to make the character concrete—for example, a miniature dragon can represent a child's temper or aggressive feelings.

After the therapist and child produce an external character to represent the child's problem, the therapist asks the child to give it a nasty name (e.g., "Trouble"). The therapist then asks the child several solution-focused questions. These "reflexive" questions (Tomm, 1987) are designed to motivate and assist the child to generate new problem-solving behaviors on his/her own. Examples of questions to evoke self-healing include "How does the problem make you feel?"; "How does the problem make your parents feel?"; "How long has the problem been pushing you around?"; and "Can you tell about the times you have not allowed the problem to get you in trouble or that you have been the boss of the problem?"

Variations

Clay Figure

A piece of clay can be formed into a dragon or monster to provide a more manageable external representation of the scary object in the child's nightmare (White & Epston, 1990).

Mad Monster Game

In this game, children are taught to see their anger as separate from themselves—for example, a "monster" that gets them into trouble. Externalizing the problem while playing this game motivates children to develop a plan to carry out a strategy to conquer their behavioral problem.

Case Illustrations

• In 1984 Australian family therapist Michael White made a simple but important discovery. While working with children who had encopresis he observed that clinical progress was enhanced when he was able to talk about the problem as if it was distinct and separate from the child. He invented the name "Sneaky Poo" to refer to the encopresis and personified it as an entity external to the child. For instance, with a particular child he might introduce the notion by asking, "What do you call the messy stuff that gets you into trouble? 'Poo?'" and "Have you ever had the experience of 'Poo' sneaking up on you and catching you unawares, say by 'popping into your pants when you were busy playing?'" If the child answers in the affirmative, White (1984) goes on to ask about the sinister influence that the character Sneaky Poo has had over the child in creating discomfort, frustration, family trouble, and so on. When the problem is clearly distinguished as being Sneaky Poo rather than the child, the complications of criticism, blame, and guilt are significantly reduced.

White followed this first line of inquiry with another set of questions about what influences the child and the family have had over the Sneaky Poo character—for instance, "Have there been times when you beat Sneaky Poo and put it in its place rather than letting Sneaky Poo beat you?" New ideas for solving the problem are then explored with the child and family—for example, "talk back" to Sneaky Poo. Therefore, the externalization technique has two components: externalizing the problem and internalizing personal agency (the ability to fight back and solve one's own externalized problem).

• Another example is that of an 8-year-old boy who was referred for initiating fights with his classmates (Butler, Guterman, & Rudes, 2009). When asked by his therapist to pick a puppet that represented his problem, the boy chose a bug puppet because his behavior was "bugging" and annoying his classmates and parents. The child used the puppet each week to remind himself to find ways to become an effective "bug buster" who was able to control his anger. After eight sessions, the boy's anger had dissipated and therapy was not needed.

Empirical Findings

Silver, Williams, Worthington, and Phillips (1998) treated 108 children ages 3–6 years with soiling problems. Half of the children received an externalization intervention and half were treated with the usual methods at the clinic. The results from the externalization group were better and compared favorably with standards from previous studies of childhood encopresis. The externalization technique was rated as much more helpful by parents at follow-up.

Applications

Externalization play has been applied to a wide range of childhood problems, including enuresis/encopresis, OCD (March & Benton, 2007; March, Mulle, & Herbal, 1994), ADHD, temper outbursts, and selective mutism.

Contraindications

The use of the externalization technique poses the risk of trivializing or minimizing serious problems in cases of domestic violence, sexual abuse, and anorexia nervosa (Freeman, Epston, & Lobovits, 1997).

References

Butler, S. J., Guterman, J., & Rudes, J. (2009). Using puppets with children in narrative therapy to externalize the problem. *Journal of Mental Health Counseling, 31*(3), 225–233.

Freeman, J., Epston, D., & Lobovits, D. (1997). *Playful approaches to serious problems.* New York: Norton.

March, J. S., with Benton, C. M. (2007). *Talking back to OCD: The program that helps kids and teens say "no way"—and parents say "way to go."* New York: Guilford Press.

March, J. S., Mulle, K., & Herbal, B. (1994). Behavioral psychotherapy for children and adolescents with obsessive–compulsive disorder: An open trial of a new protocol-driven treatment package. *Journal of the American Academy of Child and Adolescent Psychiatry, 33*(3), 333–341.

Silver, E., Williams, A., Worthington, F., & Phillips, N. (1998). Family therapy and soiling: An audit of externalizing and other approaches. *Journal of Family Therapy, 20,* 413–422.

Tomm, R. (1987). Interventive interviewing: Part II. Reflexive questioning as a means to enable self-healing. *Family Processing, 26*(2), 167–183.

White, M. (1984). Pseudo-encopresis: From avalanche to victory; from vicious to virtuous cycles. *Family Systems Medicine, 2*(2), 37–45.

White, M., & Epston, D. (1990). *Narrative means to therapeutic ends.* New York: Norton.

Winnicott, D. W. (1971). *Playing and reality.* New York: Basic Books.

18

Bibliotherapy

Books are a uniquely portable magic.
—STEPHEN KING

Introduction

Bibliotherapy dates back as far as ancient Greece where it was often used as a prescription for adults with mental illnesses (Bernstein, 1983). Samuel Crothers (1916) was the first to use the term *bibliotherapy* in reference to the use of books to help patients better understand their problems. It was not until 1936 that bibliotherapy was recommended as a form of psychotherapy for children with emotional and/or behavior problems (Bradley & Bosquet, 1936).

Carolyn Shrodes (1950) helped establish the theoretical foundation for bibliotherapy by pointing out that readers can solve their own problems by identifying with the characters in the stories. In bibliotherapy a therapist uses books about someone or something with a problem similar to that of the child. The ending of the story typically tells about adaptive ways of coping with the problem. Thus, bibliotherapy consists of using storybooks with the intent of helping the reader gain insight into and solutions for personal problems. There are two types of bibliotherapy with children. Developmental bibliotherapy aims to assist children in coping with everyday challenges. Clinical bibliotherapy seeks to help children resolve more serious emotional problems and is typically used as one part of an integrated treatment plan.

Rationale

The four main therapeutic agents in bibliotherapy are:

- *Universalization.* The child identifies with the character in a story and comes to understand that his/her situation or problem is not unique, that others have experienced the same difficulty.

- *Psychological safety.* Stories create a safe psychological distance, which allows children and adolescents to indirectly confront troublesome issues that are possibly too threatening and painful to face directly (Corr, 2004). A common feature in children's stories is the use of animal characters so as to create a distance from which children can view their own situations.

- *Problem solving.* The solution(s) utilized by the story character to a similar problem suggest to children possible ways to resolve or cope with their own difficulties.

- *Theory of mind.* Theory of mind refers to the ability to attribute mental states (e.g., beliefs, intents, desires, knowledge) to oneself and others, and to realize that the mental states of others are different from one's own. Stories help children understand the inner mental states of others, and this ability fosters empathy and social understanding.

Description

Ages

Three years and up.

Techniques

The first step is for the therapist to select a developmentally appropriate story that depicts the specific problem of the child and describes an adaptive way to deal with it. For a young child, the therapist and child read the story together (therapist reading, child turning pages, and both talking about the pictures and the story). The therapist asks questions during and after the reading, such as "What do you think the character is feeling?"; "Did you ever feel that way?"; and "What would you do in that situation?" (Gladding & Gladding, 1991). If the child responds to the book's message, follow-up activities such as drawings and doll play that relate to the text can be an effective reinforcement of the message.

Many annotated bibliographies are available to help therapists select stories for a wide variety of emotional and behavior problems of children and adolescents (Ginns-Gruenberg & Zack, 1999).

Empirical Findings

1. Although research on bibliotherapy is its infancy, Heath, Sheen, Leavy, Young, and Money (2005) report that it has proven helpful for children dealing with loss (death, parental separation), adoption, fear and anxiety, parental alcoholism, and improving self-concept.

2. In one of the first empirical studies of therapeutic storytelling, Painter, Cook, and Silverman (1999) found that it was an effective treatment with noncompliant preschoolers.

3. Klingman (1988) found that kindergarten children who were fearful of the dark showed a significant reduction in this fear after they were read stories such as *Uncle Lightfoot, Flip That Switch: Overcoming Fear of the Dark* (Coffman, 2012), in which the characters dealt effectively with the same difficulty. Children in the control group who were read neutral stories did not report a reduction in their fears.

4. Santacruz, Mendez, and Sanchez-Meca (2006) found that bibliotherapy applied at home by parents resulted in significant improvement in the darkness phobias of children ages 4–8 years.

5. After a review of the literature, Riordan and Wilson (1989) concluded that the efficacy of bibliotherapy was increased when combined with other play therapy activities.

6. Kidd and Castano (2013) found that reading literary fiction improves theory of mind in adults.

Applications

Bibliotherapy has expanded over the years to cover a wide variety of emotional and behavior problems of children. It is a particularly helpful way for children who are unable to verbalize their feelings but can identify with characters in books. It has worked well in both individual and group settings. Bibliotherapy is typically combined with other techniques within a planned therapeutic framework.

The following is a list of books we recommend for specific problems of children ages 3–13 years.

Out-of-Home Placement

Wenger, C. (1982). The suitcase story: A therapeutic technique for children in out-of-home placement. *American Journal of Orthopsychiatry*, 52(2), 353–355. Ages 6–12 years.—This story, about a suitcase that had been so many places that it was covered with stickers, portrays the many feelings of children in out-of-home placement. Through the symbolism of a suitcase, it helps these children express their feelings of anger and fears of abandonment, and to talk about their longing for permanence. It also helps foster parents understand the child's inner world.

Wilgocki, J. (2002). *Maybe Days: A Book for Children in Foster Care*. Washington, DC: American Psychological Association Press. Ages 4 years and up.—For many children in foster care, the answer to many of their questions, such as "Will this be my permanent home?" is often "Maybe." *Maybe Days* is a candid look at the issues surrounding foster care, the questions children ask, and the feelings they experience. The book, a primer for children going into foster care, also explains in children's terms the roles and responsibilities of everyone involved—parents, social workers, lawyers, and judges. As for the children, their role is simply to be a kid. The afterword contains valuable information for foster parents on ways to help the children in their care.

Death and Grief

Schwiebert, P. (2006). *Tear Soup: A Recipe for Healing After Loss.* Portland, OR: Grief Watch. Ages 8 years and up.—A family storybook that centers around Granny, a wise, old woman who has just suffered the loss of a loved one. She heads to the kitchen to make her own unique batch of "tear soup." And then she starts to cry. At first she weeps, then she sobs, eventually she wails. Slowly the pot is filled with tears as the old woman weeps away. She then stirs in precious memories of the good times and the bad times until she discovers how to find just the right blend of memories to bring comfort. By emphasizing the individual process of bereavement by making soup, Granny brings a warm and comfortable feeling to an otherwise difficult subject matter for many individuals. Winner of the 2001 Theologos Book Award, presented by the Association of Theological Booksellers.

Buscaglia, L. (1982). *The Fall of Freddie the Leaf.* Thorofare, NJ: Slack Incorporated. Ages 4–9 years.—A warm, wise, and simple story about a leaf named Freddie. The story relates how Freddie and his fellow leaves change with the passing seasons, finally falling to the ground with the winter's snow. Freddie keeps asking his wise leaf friend Daniel questions about life and death, such as "Will we all die?"; "What is the purpose of life?"; and "Where will we all go after death?" It is an inspiring allegory that illustrates the delicate balance between life and death.

Anger Management

Craver, M. M. (2011). *Chillax!: How Ernie Learns to Chill Out, Relax, and Take Charge of His Anger.* Washington, DC: Magination Press. Ages 9–13 years.—Written in an easy-to-understand comic-strip format, this is a story of a boy struggling to control his anger. He doesn't just get mad, he gets MAD! Ernie discusses his angry outbursts with a school counselor and discovers he has the power to control and calm himself. The book's lessons are evidence based and can be used by both parents and therapists. In 2012, the American Library Association's *Choice* magazine named this book an "Outstanding Academic Title."

Verdick, E. (2002). *How to Take the Grrr Out of Anger.* Minneapolis, MN: Free Spirit. Ages 8–13 years.—This book speaks directly to children with anger problems and offers them straightforward management strategies that they can use immediately. Combining information and sound advice with jokes and funny cartoons, it guides children to understand that angry feelings are normal and can be expressed in many ways—some healthy and some not. The book teaches them to become aware of and deal with angry feelings in themselves and in others. Readers learn that violence is not acceptable and that there are better, more adaptive ways to resolve conflicts. This is a kid-friendly and readable book for use in both individual and group settings.

Moser, A. (1994). *Don't Rant and Rave on Wednesdays!: The Children's Anger-Control Book.* Kansas City, MO: Landmark. Ages 4 years and up.—In this book, Moser explains the causes of anger and offers methods that can help children reduce the amount of anger they feel. He also suggests effective techniques to help young children control their behavior, even when they are very angry.

Fears and Phobias

Coffman, M. (2012). *Uncle Lightfoot, Flip That Switch: Overcoming Fear of the Dark* (2nd ed.). Footpath Press. Ages 4–8 years.—A book to help young children overcome fear of the dark through a fictional story woven around fun games. Researchers have found this book helpful in reducing fear of the dark in children when compared with a control group. In the story, Michael is afraid of the dark, and his friend, Jerome, calls him a scaredy cat. Uncle Lightfoot, a retired professor, lives on a farm nearby and knows games that can help Michael overcome his fear.

Annunziata, J. (2009). *Sometimes I'm Scared*. Washington, DC: Magination Press. Ages 5 years and up.—The book suggests easy steps children can use to cope with their everyday fears. Parents are also provided with information on the origins of fears and how to help their children understand and overcome the common fears of childhood.

Separation/Separation Anxiety

Penn, A. (1993). *The Kissing Hand*. Bronx, NY: Child Welfare League of America. Ages 3–8 years.—In this contemporary classic, Chester Raccoon seeks love and reassurance from his mother as he ventures out into the world to attend his very first day of school. His mother comforts him by kissing his paw and telling him, "Whenever you feel lonely and need a little loving from home, just press your hand to your cheek and think, 'Mommy loves you, Mommy loves you.'" The book is widely used by counselors, parents, and teachers to comfort children at times of temporary separations from home, such as entering daycare, starting school, and going to camp. It was named one of the "Top 100 Picture Books" of all time in a 2012 poll by School Library.

Karst, P. (2000). *The Invisible String*. Camarillo, CA: DeVorss & Company. Ages 4 years and up.—Children of all ages feel a great sense of comfort realizing that they are connected to love ones, especially family members living at a distance, or who have passed on, by invisible strings of love. These strings can never be broken by time, distance, or bad feelings.

Teasing/Bullying

Doleski, T. (1983). *The Hurt*. Mahwah, NJ: Paulist Press. Ages 6–8 years.—This story is about a boy whose feelings get hurt when his friend calls him a name. He holds the hurt feeling inside of him and it keeps getting bigger and bigger until he tells his father about it. By externalizing the problem, the book gives hurt feelings a concrete image that helps children understand and let go of them. It can be used in a therapeutic setting or for home reading.

Burnett, K. (1999). *Simon's Hook: A Story About Teases and Put-Downs*. Felton, CA: GR Publishing. Ages 6 years and up.—Simon has a "bad hair day" when his sister cuts out portions of his hair to remove some chewing gum. When teased by his peers, he hurries home in tears. He is consoled by his grandmother who tells him a fish story that illustrates the difficulty of providing an easy target for teasing by "biting the hook" of others.

Cohen-Posey, K. (1995). *How to Handle Bullies, Teasers and Other Meanies: A Book That Takes the Nuisance Out of Name Calling and Other Nonsense*. Highland City, FL: Rainbow Books. Ages 6 years and up.—The book gives parents, teachers, and counselors a method to help young people help themselves when confronted by annoying name calling, vicious prejudice, explosive anger, and dangerous situations. It contains more than 12 ways for handling such meanness. The book uses dozens of dialogues and practice exercises to strengthen the learning.

Divorce

Masurel, C. (2003). *Two Homes*. Somerville, MA: Candlewick Press. Ages 3–5 years.—In a simple, happy manner, the book tells about Alex, a young boy who has two homes with two sets of everything: bedrooms, bathrooms, toothbrushes, friends, and so forth. He knows he is loved by both his parents at all times no matter where he is. It focuses on what is gained rather than what is lost by a divorce. This book is recommended for helping preschool children comprehend issues related to divorce.

Brown, L., & Brown, M. (1988). *Dinosaurs Divorce: A Guide for Changing Families*. Boston: Little, Brown. Ages 3–6 years.—In an easy-to-read, comic-book-type format, this book describes the various trials and struggles of dinosaur children dealing with their dinosaur parents' divorce. It offers advice about issues such as dealing with living in two different homes, feeling you have lost your place in the family, remarriage, and stepfamilies. The book helps young children and their families cope with the confusion, misconceptions, and anxieties that are likely to arise when divorce occurs.

Trauma

Holmes, M. (2000). *A Terrible Thing Happened*. Washington, DC: Magination Press. Ages 3–8 years.—This book tells the story of a little raccoon that sees a "terrible thing." He feels much better when he is able to talk about it with the aid of a kind and understanding play therapist. The terrible thing is not identified, so the book can be used with children who have witnessed or experienced violence or trauma of any sort, including physical abuse, accidents, and natural disasters. It shows children that there is hope if they don't lock up their feelings inside, and directs them to find a caring person to listen to them.

Sheppard, C. (1998). *Brave Bart: A Story for Traumatized and Grieving Children*. Albion, MI: National Institute for Trauma and Loss in Children. Ages 4–8 years.—Bart is a little black kitten that has had a "very bad, sad, and scary thing" happen to him. He soon meets Helping Hannah, a wise cat that has aided other kittens that have also experienced a traumatic event, such as abuse or neglect. She tells him that all his (trauma) feelings are not weird but are common and normal. She helps him onto the road of healing.

Terminal Illness

Raschka, C. (2012). *The Purple Balloon*. New York: Schwartz & Wade. Ages 3 years and up.—This book offers comfort and support to children who are dying, their families, and their friends. Children tend to become aware of their impending death long before their parents want to face the possibility. The preface notes that the dying child, when given the opportunity to draw his/her feelings, will often draw a blue or purple balloon floating free on its way upward. The message of the book is that talking about dying is hard, dying is even harder, but there are many people in the child's life who can help.

Attention-Deficit/Hyperactivity Disorder

Nadeau, K., & Dixon, E. (2004). *Learning to Slow Down and Pay Attention: A Book for Kids about ADHD* (3rd ed.). Washington, DC: Magination Press. Ages 9 years and up.—This is a self-help book written especially for older children with attention-deficit disorder with hyperactivity. The authors, both clinical psychologists, clearly describe the challenges these children face, and the steps that can be taken to cope with the challenges. The straightforward text provides strategies for learning to relax, getting organized, keeping focus, completing homework, making friends, and much more. Whimsical cartoons help illustrate and reinforce the guidelines.

Stealing

Cook, J. (2012). *Ricky Sticky Fingers*. Chattanooga, TN: National Center for Youth Issues. Ages 5–10 years.—Addressing the issue of stealing, the book provides children a strategy to inhibit the urge to steal. In a light and humorous story, Ricky learns first-hand what it feels like to have something stolen from him. This experience triggers empathic feelings in him and returns the items he has stolen from others.

References

Bernstein, J. (1983). *Books to help children cope with separation and loss*. New York: Bowker.

Bradley, C., & Bosquet, E. (1936). Uses of books for psychotherapy with children. *American Journal of Orthopsychiatry, 6*, 23–31.

Corr, C. (2004). Bereavement, grief, and mourning in death-related literature for children. *Omega, 48*(4), 337–363.

Crothers, S. M. (1916). A literary classic. *Atlantic Monthly, 118*, 291–301.

Ginns-Gruenberg, D., & Zack, A. (1999). Bibliotherapy: The use of children's literature as a therapeutic tool. In C. Schaefer (Ed.), *Innovative psychotherapy techniques in child and adolescent psychotherapy* (pp. 454–489). New York: Wiley.

Gladding, S., & Gladding, C. (1991). The ABC's of bibliotherapy for school counselors. *School Counselor, 39*, 7–13.

Heath, M., Sheen, D., Leavy, D., Young, E., & Money, K. (2005). Bibliotherapy: A resource to facilitate emotional healing and growth. *School Psychology International, 26*, 563–580.

Kidd, D., & Castano, E. (2013). Reading literary fiction improves theory of mind. *Science, 342*, 377–380.

Klingman, A. (1988). Biblioguidance with kindergartners: Evaluation of a primary prevention program to reduce fear of the dark. *Journal of Clinical Child Psychology, 17*(3), 237–241.

Painter, L., Cook, J. W., & Silverman, P. (1999). The effects of therapeutic storytelling and behavioral parent training on noncompliant behavior in young boys. *Child and Family Behavior Therapy, 21*(2), 47–66.

Riordan, R., & Wilson, L. (1989). Bibliotherapy: Does it work? *Journal of Counseling and Development, 61*(9), 392–396.

Santacruz, I., Mendez, F., & Sanchez-Meca, J. (2006). Play therapy applied by parents for children with darkness phobias: Comparison of two programmes. *Child and Family Behavior Therapy, 28*(1), 19–25.

Shrodes, C. (1950). *Bibliotherapy: A theoretical and clinical-experimental study*. Unpublished doctoral dissertation, University of California, Berkeley.

Part Three

ROLE-PLAY TECHNIQUES

19

Role Play

All the world's a stage
And all the men and women merely players;
They have their exits and their entrances,
And each man in his time plays many parts.
                    —WILLIAM SHAKESPEARE

Introduction

Role play is a term used to describe a range of activities in which a person acts as if he/she was someone or something else. Role taking involves the ability to put oneself in another's place, to see things from another's point of view. It may entail an overt, observable activity or a covert, imaginative activity by a client (Corsini, 2010).

Sociodramatic play occurs when two or more children adopt roles and attempt to recreate in fantasy a real-life situation—for example, several children may assume roles as firefighters and battle a make-believe fire. Sociodramatic play has been found to significantly contribute to young children's cognitive, emotional, and social development.

Rationale

Role playing helps clients to:

- Develop a better understanding of others' viewpoints.
- Strengthen one's empathic ability and emotional intelligence.
- Gain a sense of power and control by playing the role of powerful figures.
- Acquire the necessary psychological distance to reveal one's troublesome thoughts and affects.
- Practice acting in ways that are more adaptive in real life. We tend to become what we pretend to be.

Description

Ages

Four years and up.

Techniques

The standard role-play technique involves a therapist and child assuming different roles and taking turns acting out a scenario related to the child's problem—for example, a therapist might ask a child to play out a "starting school" scenario with the therapist acting as the teacher and the child playing him/herself. The goal would be to reduce stress by making this new situation more familiar to the child and providing an opportunity to practice coping skills.

Alternately, the therapist might play the role of the child's mother giving him/her a command and asking the child to respond to it exactly as his/her mother would want the child to do. The goal here would be for the child to practice a more adaptive response.

Variations

Since there are many variations of role play, it can be adapted to almost any therapeutic situation or need. Some examples from psychodrama (Karp, Holmes, & Tauwon, 2005) include the following.

The Empty Chair

In this Gestalt therapy technique first introduced by Fritz Perls (Blom, 2006; Oaklander, 1978), a school-age child or adolescent is asked to imagine someone he/she has unresolved issues with sitting in the empty chair placed opposite of him/her, and to talk to the imagined person as if he/she is actually in the room. The client is encouraged to say to the imagined person all the things that he/she would have liked to have said in reality. This technique is often used to resolve past, unfinished, interpersonal business using present-focused pretend—for example, it might be suggested that a deceased parent is sitting in the empty chair so as to give a child the chance that was missing in real life to say goodbye. Alternately, a child might be asked to imagine his/her mother is sitting in the empty chair and to speak to her about a past, unresolved conflict between them. Children with cancer might imagine the illness is in the chair and express their feelings toward it. The technique often leads to a catharsis of pent-up feelings, both positive and negative. Some clients participate in this technique without the prop of an actual empty chair. Also, the child or adolescent might switch chairs and pretend to be the other person answering back.

Role Reversal

Role reversal refers to adopting a role the reverse of that which one normally assumes in relation to someone else. Examples include:

- Asking a child to role-play how his/her mother typically acts when he/she has done something naughty.
- Prior to a undergoing a medical procedure, the child is encouraged to play the role of doctor pretending to give the therapist an injection with actual medical equipment or medical toys. The therapist then models effective coping skills—for example, breathing or imagery. (See Chapter 3, "Medical Play.")
- *Be an expert.* A popular variation for children ages 8–12 years is for a child to pretend to be an expert on a topic related to his/her presenting problem (Hall, Kaduson, & Schaefer, 2002)—for example, a child with ADHD might play the expert on a call-in radio or TV show for parents seeking advice on how to cope with a hyperactive child.

Toy Animation

Toys naturally become animated as the child gives them an identity and voice and makes them come alive in the magical world of play. Toys, such as dolls, trucks, and puppets, can be transformed into personified characters and used by children to safely express internal needs, problems, and conflicts. Toy animation provides the safety of psychological distance and anonymity for the child and is an empowering technique that facilitates the expression of emotions, sharing of traumatic experiences, and the forming of safe therapeutic relationships. Therapists often ask children to speak as the people, animals, or objects on their fantasy play or drawings—for example, "You be that snake. What does it say?" In this way, the child can gain greater understanding of the meaning of the symbols in his/her play.

Costume and Mask Play

Costumes and masks provide further psychological distance to enable clients to express troubling thoughts and feelings. (See Chapter 20, "Costume Play," and Chapter 21, "Mask Play.")

Charades

A charade, originally a kind of riddle or guessing game, was invented in France during the 18th century. The most popular form of the game today is the acted charade in which words are acted out without any sound until they are guessed by other players in a peer or family group. Typically, you start a charade by holding both hands in front of your face, and bringing them down as if a curtain is dropped over one's face. Once your hands have passed your chin you start the charade. In therapy, the therapist writes down feeling words on pieces of paper. Group members take turns picking a slip of paper and then acting out the word written on it—using only facial expressions and body language to demonstrate the word.

For children under ages 5–6 years, the therapist or parent may need to read the words to a child. The words are kept simple for young children ages 3–6 years, such as *happy, sad, mad, grumpy, sleepy,* and *scared.* An equal number of positive and negative feelings are used. For children ages 7 years and up, more complex feelings can be used, such as *anxious, frustrated, embarrassed, proud,* and *guilty.* This technique is helpful for children who find it hard to read the emotional expression faces. A number of children, especially those on the autism spectrum struggle with recognizing the feelings they see in others.

Empirical Findings

1. Roberts and Strayer (1996) found that role-taking ability in boys ages 5–13 years was a strong predictor of empathy, which in turn was a strong predictor of prosocial behavior.

2. Iannotti (1978) reported that role-taking experiences increased altruism in 6- and 9-year-old boys.

Applications

Role-play techniques have been used with children with a wide variety of presenting problems to help them develop better coping skills to deal with challenging/stressful situations, such as teasing, and to develop empathy/compassion for others.

References

Blom, R. (2006). *The handbook of Gestalt play therapy.* London: Jessica Kingsley.

Corsini, R. (2010). *Role playing in psychotherapy.* New York: Transaction.

Hall, T., Kaduson, H., & Schaefer, C. (2002). Fifteen effective play therapy techniques. *Professional Psychology, 33*(6), 515–522.

Iannotti, R. J. (1978). Effect of role-taking experiences on role taking, empathy, altruism, and aggression. *Developmental Psychology, 14*(2), 119–124.

Karp, M., Holmes, P., & Tauwon, K. (Eds.). (2005). *The handbook of psychodrama.* London: Routledge.

Oaklander, V. (1978). *Windows to our children: A Gestalt approach to children and adolescents.* Moab, UT: Real People Press.

Roberts, W., & Strayer, J. (1996). Empathy, emotional expressiveness, and prosocial behavior. *Child Development, 67,* 449–470.

20

Costume Play

> Costumes are the first impression that you have of the character
> before they open their mouth—it really does establish who they are.
> —COLLEEN ATWOOD

Introduction

Costume play involves the use of clothing, fabric, hats, and other embellishments to play a character or type of character. Costumes are enjoyed in this country on occasion by people of all ages so they tend not to be considered too babyish by older children during play therapy. Historians believe that the use of costumes originated in Greece for the purpose of theater. Since that time, costumes have become an important part of holidays such as Halloween, Christmas, Easter, and Purim; festivals such as Mardi Gras; and sporting events in the form of mascots representing a wide variety of animals.

In recent years, "cosplay," which originated in Japan, has become a popular art form in which adult participants dress up in costumes to represent a specific character or idea. Fans of science fiction, fantasy, anime, comic book, and other genres participate in cosplay conventions. Cosplay provides participants with a creative outlet in which they express admiration for characters. They receive positive attention from audiences and peers, become part of a subculture, and have an opportunity to escape from everyday life.

Costumes also provide children with an opportunity to try on new roles, behaviors, and mannerisms. In this way, children can become whoever they want to be: a princess, pirate, nurse, teacher, cowboy, police officer, animal, or superhero. Costumes disguise one's conventional self and liberate one's personality to try out different roles and behaviors.

Rationale

Throughout the ages and different cultures, costumes have been used by people to fulfill a variety of psychological needs. Among the therapeutic powers of costume play are:

- *Self-expression.* Costumes provide children with a sense of anonymity and psychological distance that allows them to speak more freely and reveal parts of themselves they usually keep hidden. Dressed as another person, they are free to share emotions, impulses, needs, and fantasies in a spontaneous manner.

- *Self-awareness.* Costumes give children an opportunity to try on new roles and provide access to parts of their personalities that may be repressed. This fosters self-awareness and integration.

- *Positive identification.* By dressing and acting like an admired person, children form identifications that serve to enhance their own strengths. Rosenberg and Letamendi (2013) provided the following excerpt to show how qualities such as independence, self-reliance, and physical appearance inspired a cosplayer to dress up like Wonder Woman:

> It's a character I have always loved and been inspired by. Wonder Woman was a beautiful princess, but strong and independent. She took care of herself and everyone she cared about, and didn't need a prince to rescue her. Those were important qualities to me growing up in an all-woman household, just like the Amazons on Themiscrya. It didn't hurt that we were all brunettes over 5′7″ either! In Wonder Woman I saw the best qualities of my mother, and the type of woman I wanted my sister and I to become. I've always idolized her from childhood and wanted to "be" her when I grew up. (p. 14)

- *Mastery.* According to the concept of enclothed cognition, what we wear affects how we think and feel. In costume play, children have the opportunity to transform themselves, experiment with compensatory behaviors, and master developmental anxieties and fears.

- *Empathy.* Costumes disguise children's conventional self and enable them to try out different roles and behaviors. Dressing up and acting as another develops children's ability to view the world from another perspective and to empathize with thoughts and feelings of other people. In addition, this process fosters social awareness and improves social skills.

- *Positive emotion.* Costume play is enjoyable and enhances creativity, fantasy, and self-esteem. It boosts the ego and brings about a sense of well-being. When playing with others, costume play also fosters social skills.

Description

Ages

Four to 12 years.

Materials

A costume box with clothes, hats, purses, jewelry, shoes, various other props, and large pieces of fabrics in different sizes and colors facilitate projective play and character acting.

Techniques

Costume play can be used as a directive or nondirective technique in play therapy, depending on the needs of the child. Dress-up play is an ideal intervention for preschool children whose play centers around pretend. In addition, school-age children, ages 8–12 years enjoy costume props to engage in role play (Marcus, 1993). Children are especially drawn to specific costumes to enact characters such as police officer, firefighter, superhero, princess, teacher, and adult.

Variations

Identification Role Play

This technique helps children identify with and internalize the qualities of an admired individual or character. Therapists and parents can use the technique to help children overcome insecurities, fears, and anxieties—for example, the parent of a child who is afraid of the dark might be advised to use identification role play by dressing the child in superhero pajamas at bedtime. Therapists can do the same by providing a variety of costumes to help children attain a sense of empowerment. Taylor, Carlson, and Maring (2004) described a case of a 5-year-old boy who engaged in costume play after experiencing a frightening thunderstorm. When the boy impersonated a character he called "Super Lightning Bolt Adam" by wearing a cape and mask, he spoke and behaved with confidence and power.

Crown Game: On Being Kings and Queens

Gold (2003) introduced this technique as a projective tool to gain entry into children's thoughts, feelings, and values. The child is first engaged in a fantasy play in which the therapist says, "We are assembled before the Royal Court in the great drawing room. We are in the process of crowning the next Queen/King. There are maidens in fine gowns everywhere, and all the knights are wearing their armor." The child is then given a crown, asked to put it on his or her head and told, "You are King/Queen for this moment. What would please you the most, your highness?" (p. 350).

Empirical Findings

1. Karniol, Galili, and Shtilerman (2011) examined factors that contribute to preschoolers' ability to delay gratification. The researchers found that preschool children told about Superman's ability to delay gratification while wearing capes were able to delay gratification longer than preschoolers not wearing capes. In another study, the same researchers found that preschoolers who pretended to be Superman were able to delay gratification longer than preschoolers who watched a Superman video.

2. Adam and Galinsky (2012) examined the concept of "enclothed cognition" and found that young adults who donned a lab coat performed better on a sustained attention task than others who merely saw a lab coat on a desk. Other studies have found that a football team dressed in black uniforms act more aggressive than teams dressed in lighter-colored uniforms.

Applications

Costume play can help verbally reticent children become more expressive in play therapy. It can also empower children to overcome anxieties and fearfulness—for example, a superhero costume might encourage children with selective mutism to speak.

References

Adam, H., & Galinsky, A. (2012). Enclothed cognition. *Journal of Experimental Social Psychology, 48*(4), 918–925.

Gold, D. C. (2003). The crown game: On being kings and queens. In H. G. Kaduson & C. E. Schaefer (Eds.), *101 favorite play therapy techniques* (Vol. 3, pp. 349–351). Lanham, MD: Jason Aronson.

Karniol, R., Galili, L., & Shtilerman, D. (2011). Why superman can wait: Cognitive self-transformation in the delay of gratification paradigm. *Journal of Clinical Child and Adolescent Psychology, 40*(2), 307–317.

Marcus, I. (1993). Costume play therapy. In C. Schaefer & D. Cangelosi (Eds.), *Play therapy techniques* (pp. 91–100). Northvale, NJ: Jason Aronson.

Rosenberg, R. S., & Letamendi, A. M. (2013). Expressions of fandom: Findings from a psychological survey of cosplay and costume wear. *Intensities: The Journal of Cult Media*, pp. 9–18. Retrieved from *www.drrobinrosenberg.com/resources/Cosplay-Expressions%20of%20Fandom.pdf*.

Taylor, M., Carlson, S., & Maring, B. (2004). The characteristics and correlates of fantasy in school-age children: Imaginary companions, impersonation, and social understanding. *Developmental Psychology, 40*(6), 1173–1187.

21

Mask Play

Man is least himself when he talks in his own person. Give him a
mask, and he will tell you the truth.

—OSCAR WILDE

Introduction

Masks include any object used to cover the face for ritual practices, entertainment,
disguise, make-believe, or protection. Masks have been used throughout history
by cultures around the world and date back as early as 7000 B.C.E. African tribes
used masks in rituals to communicate with ancestral and animal spirits, to scare
enemies, and as symbols of various attributes. Inuit tribes in America wore masks
to unite with ancestors and to exorcise evil spirits from the sick. Ancient Egyptians
used death masks so that the soul could recognize the body and return to it.

Masks have also been used as a way to change identity and assume a new persona since ancient times. They were used as a form of disguise in Venice during the
Middle Ages. In contemporary societies, masks are used for festivals such as Mardi
Gras, New Year's celebrations, and social protests. They are also used for protection by welders, firefighters, and medical and dental professionals, among others.

Rationale

In therapy, masks are commonly used as a projective tool and form of self-expression. Landy (1986) proposed that masks can also be used to represent two sides of
a conflict or problem, to express one's identity in a group, to explore dreams and
imagery, and to characterize social roles.

Mask making commonly incorporates the Jungian concepts of persona and
shadow. According to Jung, the persona is the appearance we present to the world
in order to adapt to the demands of society. It includes social roles, mannerisms,

the clothes we choose to wear, and so on. The persona enables individuals to make impressions upon others and at the same time, it conceals their true nature. Jung wrote, "One could say, with little exaggeration, that the persona is that which in reality one is not, but which oneself as well as others think one is" (Storr, 1983, p. 422). The shadow, according to Jung's theory, is the negative part of our personality that we do not show the world because it contains qualities that are not compatible with social demands. Jung believed that the shadow epitomizes all the things that we refuse to acknowledge about ourselves, but which continuously affect us either directly or indirectly. Jung believed that "everyone carries a shadow, and the less it is embodied in the individual's conscious life, the blacker and denser it is" (Storr, 1983, p. 88).

Jung also believed that acquiring self-knowledge involves understanding the relationship between the true self and the persona he/she shows the world. In Jungian theory, a major goal of treatment is to integrate the persona with the real self and to bring the shadow into consciousness. Masks are ideal for these purposes because they allow individuals to externalize parts of the self. Landy (1985) wrote:

> In therapeutic mask work, then, the mask is used as a projective technique to separate one part of the self from another. The masked part, the persona, being stylized and dramatic, provides a measure of distance from the person. Through the work with the persona, the person comes to see his dilemma more clearly. The therapeutic masquerade or drama of masks aims to unmask the self through masking a part of the self that has been repressed or seen dimly by the client. (p. 51)

Additional therapeutic benefits of mask play include:

• *Self-expression.* Masks provide a make-believe tool that allows children to speak anonymously. This gives them freedom to express feelings, needs, and experiences in a candid, yet disguised manner.

• *Safety.* Masks provide immediate psychological distance and a sense of safety for the wearer. Gallo-Lopez and Schaefer (2005) note that even simple coverings, such as sunglasses, are transformational and equip children with a ready disguise and source of safety.

• *Therapeutic alliance.* Mask making is an enjoyable activity that is familiar and engaging. It can be used in the early stages of treatment as an ice-breaker to enhance comfort and establish a trusting relationship with the therapist.

• *Creative thinking.* Mask making involves planning, organization, and creativity. Children determine the kind of mask they wish to make, what it will convey, and the materials used to make it. This process involves problem solving and fosters flexible thinking. In addition, the reward of creating a one-of-a-kind mask fosters pride and a sense of self-esteem.

• *Projective play.* With masks and other face coverings, children can be whomever they want to be. This allows them to openly express memories, fears, desires, needs, and fantasies—for example, in sunglasses children can become a famous actor or a wanted robber.

Description

Ages

Four years and up.

Materials

Depending on the age and developmental level of the child, therapists may choose to provide store-bought masks or materials for one to be made. Very young children can make simple masks with store-bought blank masks, paper plates, or oval pieces of construction paper with eyeholes. Older children, adolescents, and adults can make more sophisticated masks from cardboard, plaster of Paris, papier-mâché, or rigid wrap cloths. It is important that the therapist provide ample time and a diverse selection of embellishments to enhance creativity and self-expression. These would include a variety of paints, markers, feathers, ribbons, beads, jewels, and stickers.

Techniques

Inside–Outside Masks (Kurczek, 2001)

In this technique, children make a collage on the outside of a mask, using cut-out pictures and words from magazines representing how the outside world sees them. They then make a second collage on the inside of the mask, using cut-out pictures and words representing who they are inside at the deepest level. The inside mask aids clients to discover the difference between their persona (or false selves) and who they are at the core.

Grief Mask

Children often put on a brave front and hide their true feelings after a loss. The grief mask is a tool that helps them express these emotions. Using clay or papier-mâché, children ages 6 years and up mold a mask from scratch, forming it in whatever shape they desire. They then decorate the outside of the mask with colors and embellishments that represent how they truly feel. Materials such as paint, ribbon, foam, markers, feathers, gems, and glitter are provided to enhance expression of , emotions (Grief Masks & Sculpture, n.d; Imhoff, Vance, & Quackenbush, n.d.). In a variation of this technique, children decorate the inside of the mask to convey how they feel, and the outside to convey what they show the world.

Possible-Selves Mask

The idea for this technique comes from the possible-selves concept proposed by Markus and Nurius (1986). In this technique, teens create masks representing their past self (where they have been), their present self (where they are now), and their future self (who they want to be). This activity (Brumleve, 2010) allows adolescents to explore identity issues and gives them an opportunity to experiment and try on one or more potential future selves. Looking at the future self promotes goal setting, self-improvement, malleability, and personal growth (Oyserman, Bybee, & Terry, 2006).

Family Role-Play Masks

In a family therapy session, the therapist asks a family member to wear a mask depicting the face of another family member (e.g., child wears a "father mask") and then role-plays how that person reacted to a specific family event (e.g., a sibling fight; Baptiste, 1989). Alternately, each family member could be asked to stimulate family discussion by selecting a mask to represent the dark side of their personality or a quality/feature they would like more of.

Empirical Findings

1. Pollaczek and Homefield (1954) proposed that role-playing with masks is a useful technique for children and adults with a negative self-image. In working with children, they found that masks served to decrease stuttering and increase nonverbal expression.

2. Zhong, Bohns, and Gino (2010) found that wearing sunglasses altered people's sense of anonymity—that is, people in sunglasses admitted to feeling more anonymous than those wearing clear eyeglasses.

3. Miller and Rowold (1979) found that children wearing Halloween masks were more likely to break a rule than children not wearing a mask. In this study, 58 children were told that they could take two pieces of candy from a bowl and were then left alone. Results showed that 62% of the children in masks broke the two-candy limit, compared with 37% of those whose faces were visible. The researchers propose that masks serve to elicit a state of anonymity, which leads to lowered restraints on behavior.

Applications

Masks are a valuable therapeutic technique to facilitate self-expression in children. Because they allow individuals to externalize and distance from problems, they are especially helpful for treating anxious and inhibited children who have difficulties expressing emotions; individuals with histories of loss, separation, and trauma; and adolescents struggling with identity issues. Baptise (1989) noted that masks are also helpful for treating high-conflict families. Masks enable family members to see one another in a new way and correct distorted and rigid perceptions. He wrote:

> Through involvement with this technique, family members learn to use humor and play creatively to "unmask" and confront each other as persons by getting from behind the personal mask each has created and wears as a defense against the other. (p. 46)

References

Baptise, D. A. (1989). Using masks as therapeutic aids in family therapy. *Journal of Family Therapy, 11*, 45–58.

Brumleve, E. (2010). Expressive mask making for teens: Beginning insights. Alexandria, VA: American Art Therapy Association. Retrieved from *www.arttherapy.org/upload/News&Info/ExpressiveMaskMakingForTeens.pdf*.

Gallo-Lopez, L., & Schaefer, C. E. (2005). *Play therapy with adolescents*. Northvale, NJ: Jason Aronson.

Grief Masks & Sculpture. (n.d.). Connect with your soul. Retrieved from *www.recover-from-grief.com/grief-masks.html*.

Imhoff, B. A., Vance, K. V., & Quackenbush, A. (n.d.). Helping bereaved children: 20 activities for processing grief. Retrieved from *www.allohiocc.org/Resources/Documents/AOCC%202012%20Session%2062.pdf*.

Kurczek, T. A. (2001). Inside–outside masks. In H. G. Kaduson & C. E. Schaefer (Eds.), *101 more favorite play therapy techniques* (pp. 70–74). Northvale, NJ: Jason Aronson.

Landy, R. J. (1985). The image of the mask: Implications for theatre and therapy. *Journal of Mental Imagery, 9*(4), 43–56.

Landy, R. J. (1986). *Drama therapy: Concepts and practices*. Springfield, IL: Charles Thomas.

Markus, H., & Nurius, P. (1986). Possible selves. *American Psychologist, 41*(9), 954–969.

Miller, F. G., & Rowold, K. L. (1979). Halloween masks and deindividuation. *Psychological Reports, 44*(2), 422.

Oyserman, D., Bybee, D., & Terry, K. (2006). Possible selves and academic outcomes: How and when possible selves impel action. *Journal of Personality and Social Psychology, 91*(1), 188–204.

Pollaczek, P. P., & Homefield, H. D. (1954). The use of masks as an adjunct to role playing. *Mental Hygiene, 38*, 299–304.

Storr, A. (1983). *The essential Jung*. Princeton, NJ: Princeton University Press.

Zhong, C.-B., Bohns, V. K., & Gino, F. (2010). Good lamps are the best police: Darkness increases dishonesty and self-interested behavior. *Psychological Science, 21*(3), 311–314.

22

Superhero Play

Children wear their Spider-Man T-shirts, sleep on their Buzz
Lightyear pillows, and take the latest superhero vitamin, all in an
effort to achieve power.

—PATTY SCANLON

Introduction

American comic books originated in 1933 and became a favorite pastime with the
introduction of Superman in 1938. Within a year after his introduction, Superman
had a comic book named after him, which sold over one million copies each issue.
In 1939, other superheroes joined Superman: the Human Torch, the Sub-Mariner,
the Flash, and Wonder Woman. During this time, superheroes were especially
appealing to teenage boys. With qualities such as intelligence, kindness, power,
and a value for righting wrongs and preventing catastrophes, they represented ide-
alized versions of boy-/manhood. Many early comic book writers were young Jew-
ish men, aware of their status as outsiders in America. Most superheroes they created were outsiders with special abilities that often battled superpowers, a theme
that resonated with adolescents.

Bender and Laurie (1941) were intrigued by children's enthusiasm about
superheroes and argued that their mythological quality makes them a useful tool
for helping children address psychological difficulties and real-life dangers. Bender
and Laurie likened the comic strip to "folklore of the times, spontaneously given to
and received by children, serving at the same time as a means of helping them solve
the individual and sociological problems appropriate to their own lives" (p. 54).
The children Bender and Laurie treated used fantasy play inspired by Superman to
address issues of personal protection, as an ego ideal, and a problem solver.

Many years later, Lawrence and Jewett (2002) expanded Bender and Laurie's ideas about superheroes and highlighted their key characteristics. They noted that superheroes originate outside of the community or society they must save, have secret or dual identities, tend to be selfless and idealistic loners, value justice, show restraint for revenge, and are morally infallible. Superheroes also have superhuman powers and do not cause undue injury to others, even archenemies. "The superhero's aim is unerring, his fists irresistible, and his body incapable of suffering fatal injury" (p. 47).

Rationale

Rubin (2007) argued that the central issues of superheroes relate to the struggles children and adolescents experience and provide a framework for superhero play in therapy. These include themes related to the origin story, transformation, villain, dual or secret identity, family dynamics, superpowers and fatal flaws, science and magic, and costumes. Just as superheroes have origin stories, children attempt to understand their own origins. Just as superheroes are transformed by situations beyond their control, children are changed by abuse, loss, and trauma. Like superheroes, children have archenemies they must cope with and battles they must overcome. Similar to the challenges of having dual identities in superheroes, children struggle to work out internal conflicts. Whether transformed by science or magic, superheroes rarely fit in. Similarly, children struggle with identity and belonging issues (Rubin, 2007). These similarities make superhero play an ideal way for working with children and adolescents and provide a number of therapeutic benefits:

- *Power.* The vulnerability of young children leads to their desire for superpowers. Identifying with the strengths and powers of superheroes can be transformative and instill in them the courage to overcome their fears, face challenges, and master problems.

- *Identity formation.* Identification with superhero mythology can help children incorporate superhero traits into their personality and lives.

- *Overcoming resistance.* Superhero play is a great way to engage children in treatment. Children naturally enjoy role-playing superhero themes, discussing movies, storytelling, playing with action figures, and creating superheroes with clay or other art materials. Young children also enjoy dressing like superheroes and using miniature figures to enact adventures. In addition, the histories, challenges, and personalities of superheroes resonate with adolescents and provide a way for them to address their own issues.

- *Fantasy.* Through superhero fantasy play, children try out new roles and explore new ways to cope with difficulties. This increases their imaginations and creative problem-solving ability.

Description

Ages

Four to 12 years.

Superhero play is useful in both individual and group counseling and can be implemented in a number of ways depending on the age, needs, and interests of the child. These include dress up/fantasy play, drawings, handouts, art activities, comic book/movie discussions, role playing, storytelling, sand tray play, and computer/telephone apps. Superhero play can be also be used in milieu therapy (Robertie, Weidenbrenner, Barrett, & Poole, 2007) and hypnotherapeutic interventions such as breathing exercises, yoga, and chanting (Burte, 2007).

Technique

Stress Busting

Provide the child with a costume of a favorite or familiar superhero and the opportunity for superhero play in session and/or at home. Remind the child of the personal qualities of the superhero, such as courage, strength, and resiliency. During superhero play some children may become overexcited and need clear limits set and enforced on aggressive/destructive behaviors. When the child has become confident in the role of a superhero, encourage the child to wear his/her superhero costume when anxious at home, such as to bed to overcome the fear of the dark.

Variations

Shazam

This technique by Cangelosi (2001) is useful for children of all ages. The child uses clay or art materials of his/her choice to create a "messenger" friend (animal, alien, cartoon character, etc.) that will help him/her solve problems. While the child creates the messenger, a discussion takes place regarding the problems that it will help with. When the messenger is completed, the therapist asks the child to close his/her eyes and imagine it. The therapist then explains that Shazam (or whatever name the child chooses for the messenger) will be invisible to everyone except the child but will remain with the child at all times to remind him/her about options for dealing with the problems discussed.

Superhero Drawing

First ask the child if he/she could have superhero powers, what would they be? Then suggest a self-drawing with these powers. Then discuss what these powers are and how the child might use them in real life. Point out how the child's natural strengths can be as effective as superpowers.

The Power Animal: Internalizing a Positive Symbol of Strength

This technique, introduced by Hickey (2001), is for children of all ages. The therapist shows the child pictures of a large variety of animals and asks the child to choose one that appeals to him/her. The therapist then asks the child to construct the chosen animal in clay or to make a mask with the animal face on it. The therapist follows the child's lead. Eventually, the therapist will ask the child to imagine what the animal might do in certain situations and how it might solve a specific problem. By regularly consulting with the animal, the therapist will help the child move deeper into an internalization of the strengths and attributes the child projects onto the animal. This technique is useful for children with low self-esteem and difficulties with problem-solving and social skills.

Super Me

Nickerson (2001) developed this storytelling technique for children ages 4–9 years to facilitate the termination process. The child describes the qualities that he/she would give to a superhero and creates one with art materials, giving it a costume, weapon, and name. The therapist then tells a story about the child and the superhero solving a problem together. The goal is for the child to internalize the strengths of the superhero. The child takes the superhero creation home at the last session as a reminder of his/her strengths and accomplishments in therapy.

Comic-Book-Making Kits

Tomy Toys produced this Mighty Men and Monster Maker kit for children ages 6 years and up. It contains tiles showing legs, torsos, and heads that can be mixed and matched to create a superhero. The child places a piece of paper over the tiles, closes the lid of the carrier to hold the paper in place, and then uses a crayon to rub over the tiles to create a superhero or villain. Crayola Story Studio Comic Maker, for children ages 6 years and up, provides an online access code that allows children to morph photos of themselves into Spiderman and insert them into a comic adventure. In addition, handouts can be made by the therapist with six to eight blank grids for the child to draw scenes of a superhero story.

Superhero Parent

The child's parent wears a superhero cape or costume on occasion and models acting brave and strong during a stressful life event (e.g., a medical procedure).

Empirical Findings

   1. Chung and de Silva (2013) found that self-transformation through pretend play affected the executive functioning performance in preschoolers. Thirty-two preschoolers participated in their study and were divided into two groups. Children in the self-transformation group were given a cape that was described as having special powers, enabling the wearer to play games well. Children in the control group were given the same cape but were told that it was part of the game. The children then participated in three different executive functioning tasks: two response inhibition tasks and one attention-shifting task. Children in the self-transformation group had significantly higher combined response inhibition scores than children in the control group and higher scores on the task requiring attention shifting.

2. Parsons and Howe (2013) report that preschool boys who engaged in two superhero play sessions (vs. boys who played with generic toys) exhibited significantly more prosocial behaviors, whereas there were more disruptive behaviors in the generic toy sessions.

3. In her doctoral dissertation, Elizabeth Robinson (2014) found that superhero knowledge was significantly and positively related to moral judgment in fifth-grade boys. The data indicated that the boys were able to see beyond violence and fighting to see the positive outcomes of superheroes helping people, fighting crime, and doing the right thing.

4. Karniol and colleagues (2011) asked a group of Superman-caped preschoolers and a group of uncaped preschoolers to delay gratification. Caped children delayed longer, especially when instructed about Superman's delay-relevant qualities.

Contraindications

This technique is not appropriate for children with a weak grasp on reality who could lose their sense of self in the play by assuming the identity of a superhero character and acting out accordingly.

Applications

Superhero play is an ideal way to engage children of all ages and diagnostic categories in treatment. It is especially useful for children with issues related to fears, phobias, trauma, adoption, and attachment issues. In addition, superhero play is a great tool for teaching compassion, kindness, justice, "taking the high road," and social skills.

References

Bender, L., & Laurie, R. (1941). The effect of comic books on the ideology of children. *American Journal of Orthopsychiatry, 11*(3), 540–550.

Burte, J. M. (2007). Hypnosis and superheroes. In L. Rubin (Ed.), *Using superheroes in counseling and play therapy* (pp. 271–292). New York: Springer.

Cangelosi, D. (2001). Shazam. In H. G. Kaduson & C. E. Schaefer (Eds.), *101 more favorite play therapy techniques* (pp. 455–457). Northvale, NJ: Jason Aronson.

Chung, K. K., & de Silva, A. D. (2013). Effects of a pretend play intervention on executive functioning tasks. Wellesley College Digital Scholarship and Archive Student Library Research Awards Archives. Retrieved from *http://repository.wellesley.edu/cgi/viewcontent.cgi?article=1004&context=library_award*.

Hickey, D. A. (2001). The power animal technique: Internalizing a positive symbol of strength. In H. G. Kaduson & C. E. Schaefer (Eds.), *101 more favorite play therapy techniques* (pp. 451–454). Northvale, NJ: Jason Aronson.

Karniol, R., Galili, L., Shtilerman, D., Naim, K., Manjoch, H., & Silverman, R. (2011). Why Superman can wait: Cognitive self-transformation in the delay of gratification paradigm. *Journal of Clinical Child and Adolescent Psychology*, 40(2), 307–317.

Lawrence, J. S., & Jewett, R. (2002). *The myth of the American superhero*. Cambridge, UK: Erdmans.

Nickerson, E. (2001). Super me! In H. G. Kaduson & C. E. Schaefer (Eds.), *101 more favorite play therapy techniques* (pp. 25–28). Northvale, NJ: Jason Aronson.

Parsons, A., & Howe, N. (2013). "This is Siderman's mask." "No, it's Green Goblin's": Shared meanings during boys' pretend play with superhero and generic toys. *Journal of Research in Childhood Education*, 27(2), 190–207.

Robertie, K., Weidenbrenner, R., Barrett, L., & Poole, R. (2007). A super milieu: Using superheroes in the residential treatment of adolescents with sexual behavior problems. In L. C. Rubin (Ed.), *Using superheroes in counseling and play therapy* (pp. 143–168). New York: Springer.

Robinson, E. (2014). *The influence of superhero characters on moral judgment in school-age children*. Doctoral dissertation, Alfred University, New York.

Rubin, L. C. (2007). Introduction: Look, up in the sky! An introduction to the use of superheroes in psychotherapy. In L. C. Rubin (Ed.), *Using superheroes in counseling and play therapy* (pp. 143–168). New York: Springer.

23

Puppet Play

Introduction

Puppet play is a popular play technique that helps children express feelings, reenact anxiety-laden events, try out new, more adaptive behaviors, and overcome inhibitions. The fact that puppetry has survived from man's early beginnings to the present day gives proof of its inherent strength and wide appeal. Puppets are more vivid, more alive, and more interesting than dolls, and can be manipulated without much practice.

The first and most extensive use of puppets in psychotherapy was by Bender and Woltmann (1936) at the Children's Psychiatry Ward of Bellevue Hospital in New York City. Adult puppeteers presented puppet shows to assist the children to identify with and project their problems onto the puppet characters that in the end found solutions to their problems. A group discussion based on the shows followed each performance. Hand puppets were used because "they are more direct in their actions, more convincing in their movements, and capable of more aggression than string marionettes" (Bender & Woltmann, 1936, p. 343). A hand puppet consists of a three-dimensional head attached to a cloth body.

Rationale

The variety of therapeutic benefits from puppet play span many theoretical orientations and include:

• *Projection.* Children identify with puppets. Puppet play enables them to project their thoughts, feelings, and needs that they are unable or unwilling to express in words (Jenkins & Beckh, 1942). Children find it easier to reveal their inner world through the medium of a "third person"—that is, a puppet (Cassell,

1965). If the puppet says or does something wrong, the puppet is at fault, not the child. Thus, puppets provide a safe psychological distance for a child to express troublesome experiences, thoughts, and emotions—for example, a child may use puppets to act out scenes observed or experienced at home, such as child or spouse abuse (Bromfield, 1995).

• *Displacement.* A child may safely express hostile feelings toward a parent onto a puppet without the risk of retaliation.

• *Ego boosting.* The complete control a child has over a puppet expands his/ her ego by giving a sense of mastery.

• *Increased interest in learning.* Since puppet plays makes learning interesting and fun for children, they can facilitate the learning of new skills, such as problem solving and social skills.

• *Abreactive healing.* A stressful life experience can be reenacted in puppet play so as to enable a child to have a cathartic release of feelings and to develop of a sense of mastery over the stressful event (Waelder, 1933).

Description

Ages

Five to 11 years.

Materials

A collection of 15–20 soft, hand puppets for individual therapy; 25–30 for group or family therapy. The collection should include wild and domestic animals, human figures, and symbolic characters, such as dragons, devils, and fairies.

A wide variety of puppet play techniques have proven helpful for assessment and therapy with children. A selection of popular techniques follow.

Puppet Assessment Techniques

Structured Interview of a Child (Irwin, 1993)

• Step 1: Present the child with a collection of 15–20 easy-to-manipulate hand puppets representing a broad range of psychological and social characteristics (e.g., aggression, nurturance, timidity).

• Step 2: As a warm-up, ask the child to introduce the selected puppet to you by saying its name, age, and gender. A central assumption is that children tend to choose puppets that have significant meaning for them. The puppets often represent parts of their personality (e.g., a mouse puppet for the timidity in them), or the character of people around them (e.g., a witch puppet as the personification of a mean mother figure).

- Step 3: Ask the child to tell a made-up story with the puppet(s) behind a puppet stage or overturned table.

- Step 4: When the puppet show is over, the therapist interviews the puppet characters(s) and then the child to elicit additional information about the characters and why they acted as they did. In the imaginary stories of children, certain themes will likely appear as the child projects his/her own life stories onto the puppet. This postshow discussion helps the therapist more fully understand the personal meaning of the puppet show for the child.

Family Puppet Interview (Irwin & Malloy, 1975)

In this approach, the therapist presents a collection of 25–30 puppets to the family members. Family members are asked to select one or two puppets to help tell their piece of a story. The family then decides together on a story in which each of their puppets has a part. A story should have a beginning, middle, and end. Many families decide to tell a well-known fairytale that all family members know. The family then presents the story they have developed—with the therapist as the audience. After the story the therapist interviews each of the puppet characters about their role in and motive for their actions in the story. Finally, the therapist encourages the family members to discuss the puppet show, including their thoughts and feelings about the characters, and any real-life similarities. The "group puppet interview" developed by Bratton and Ray (1999) applies this technique to members of a child therapy group.

Wittenborn, Faber, Harvey, and Thomas (2006) used the family puppet interview with a family consisting of a mom, dad, and 8-year-old daughter. The mom chose a cat puppet, the girl a puppy, and the dad a grim-looking gorilla. In their story the gorilla tries to take control of the situation by telling the cat and puppy what to do. The puppy runs away and the cat does not know what to do.

This is just one case example of how family puppet plays can provide valuable information about family dynamics (Gil, 2015; Gil, Sobol, & Bailey, 2005), such as:

- The level of cooperation, involvement, and organization displayed by the family and the roles they assumed in completing this task.
- The ability of the family to reach agreement on the story and the way it was reached.
- The degree of enjoyment exhibited in engaging in this task.
- The level of insight—for example, seeing the play as a metaphor for their own reality.

Berkeley Puppet Interview (Measelle, Ablow, Cowan, & Cowan, 1998)

This is a structured interview of young (ages 4–8 years) children's perceptions of the family environment, school performance, peer relationships, and symptomatology. The therapist conducts the interview with two dog puppets, Iggy and Ziggy, that ask the child to indicate which of two opposing statements is most like him/her. The two statements reflect the positive and negative ends of two different behaviors or attributes (e.g., "I tease other kids" and "I don't tease other kids. What about you?"; "My mom yells at me a lot" and "My mom doesn't yell at me a lot"; "My dad is in a bad mood a lot" and "My dad is not in a bad mood a lot"; "I like to read" and "I don't like to read"). This assessment tool is particularly suitable for nonverbal, shy, and selectively mute children since the child can either respond nonverbally by pointing, or talk in the third person by using a puppet to respond to the interviewer's questions.

Puppet Therapy Techniques

Using a Puppet to Create a Symbolic Client

A puppet can be used as a pretend client who needs help with a similar problem as the child's (e.g., being bullied, feeling sad, or afraid; Narcavage, 1997). This allows the child to separate him/herself from the situation and look at it through a more objective eye, which can help find a solution to the problem. Thus, a therapist might show a child, ages 4–8 years, a puppet that has a similar problem and encourage the child to help comfort the puppet and subsequently give the puppet advice (with the therapist's coaching) about how to solve the problem (e.g., ignoring or staying calm when teased). By shifting attention to the puppet, the child gains psychological distance from the problem, which increases the child's engagement in addressing the problem.

For example, a 3-year-old boy had a recurrent biting problem and was in danger of being expelled from day care. The therapist introduced the boy to Leo, an alligator puppet with a big mouth. He told the boy that Leo had a big problem in that he keeps biting people, like this, and it hurts and people get so upset that it ends up making Leo feel very bad. After listening intently, the held the alligator puppet and bit his own arm with it and yelled "Ouch!" When asked if he had any ideas to help Leo stop biting, the boy ran to get the toy telephone and called Leo. He said to Leo, "Come home right now!" When Leo arrived, the boy told him he could not bite people but he could bite a toy. The therapist mentioned that Leo cries big crocodile tears after he bites because he first wants to bite but is sad that he hurts people and people are mad at him. The boy kept Leo at his side throughout the session.

As another example, if a child is very fearful on entering the playroom for the first time, the therapist might introduce a "Mr. Bear" puppet and have the puppet cover its eyes out of fear. The therapist would then say to "Mr. Bear" that she knows how scared he is to come to a new place with a grown-up he didn't know. She would reassure Mr. Bear that he is in a safe place, with a safe person who will not let anything bad happen to him or the child client.

Therapist's Friend Puppet

Select a puppet to be your friend during a session with an aggressive child. When the child acts mean to you, your puppet would react by saying such supportive statements as "Wow, that was a hurtful thing to say!" and "I don't think it's OK to talk to an adult like that." Indirect feedback from a puppet is easier for a child to take than direct therapist confrontation.

Externalizing the Child's Problem

Externalization is a narrative therapy technique to objectify, and at times, to personify in the form of a puppet the problem the child is experiencing. The goal is for clients to see themselves as separate from their problems (see Chapter 17, "Externalization Play"). Butler, Guterman, and Rudes (2009) describe a case involving an 8-year-old boy who frequently fought in the classroom. When asked to choose a puppet that most closely resembled his problem of annoying others, he selected a bug puppet because his fighting behavior was annoying (bugging) others.

Puppet Stress Inoculation

In this puppet modeling technique (Shapiro, 1995), the therapist introduces a puppet that had experienced a stressor identical to the one the child will undergo, such as starting school, a medical procedure, or fear of the dark. The goal of this technique is to reduce the unknown aspects of a stressor and demonstrate useful coping techniques. After explaining that the puppet just experienced the same stressor that the child will, the therapist has the puppet show and tell coping strategies it used while undergoing the stressful event (e.g., positive imagery, deep breathing). The child is encouraged to ask the puppet any questions he/she wishes about the event.

Group Mascot

In the first session of a play therapy group Pedro-Carroll and Jones (2005) have found it helpful for the therapist to introduce to the group a "shy" puppet (perhaps hidden in a bag) that is anxious about what to expect from the group. The therapist then asks the group members to help the puppet feel accepted and comfortable in the group. They have found that group members typically respond with help-ful suggestions, such as "Let's tell him our names and what we'll be doing in the group." This often leads to a group discussion of common interests, favorite foods, and so on. The puppet also shares personal interests/problems and assumes the role of group mascot.

Mutual Puppet Show

First, the child and therapist each select a puppet or two to animate. Then the child is asked to begin a puppet show in which the child and therapist take turns telling the puppet story. The therapist uses his/her turn to present a more adaptive solution to the story or a positive reframing of the motives or behaviors of child's puppet character (Hawkey, 1951).

Group Puppet Charades

Each child in the group is given a specific emotion or situation to act out with the puppet without talking. The other group members are asked to guess what the emotion or situation is.

Free Puppet Play

The child is given the freedom to spontaneously select, animate, and direct the actions of a puppet or two as he/she wishes. The therapist serves as the audience and asks the child to introduce the puppet(s) before using them to act out a story. The therapist can later interview a puppet character or the child to gain further clarification of the meaning of the puppet story.

Puppet "Talk Show"

The goal of this technique is to give members of a child play therapy group a way to bond by getting to know one another better. Each child is asked to choose a puppet from a collection of realistic human and fantasy puppets displayed on a table or on the floor. Each child's puppet is then interviewed using a "talk show" format. The therapist serves as the "talk show host" and the other children are the audience members who take turns asking each child's puppet personal questions, such as "What is your favorite food?" and "What makes you mad?" Each group member decides to have the selected puppet represent him/herself or to create a fantasy character that answers the questions. The puppets provide psychological distance for the children to facilitate the disclosure of their inner world of thoughts, feel-ings, and desires.

Puppet Story Character

The use of a puppet to represent a character in a therapeutic story the therapist is telling helps to bring the tale to life. The child can ask the puppet about what happens next in the story as well as give the puppet advice on how to handle situations in the story.

Empirical Findings

1. Carter and Mason (1998) found that it is most beneficial to provide 15–20 puppets for children. Providing too few puppets will not allow for projection of internal experiences and too many puppets will likely overwhelm the child.

2. Working with hospitalized children undergoing cardiac catheterization, Cassell (1965) found that they were able to express their emotions about the procedure through puppets. Consequently, they were less emotionally upset during the procedure and more willing to return to the hospital for further treatment.

3. Gronna, Serna, Kennedy, and Prater (1999) used puppet script training to teach social skills of greeting and initiating/responding to conversations to a preschool child with visual impairments. This single case study, using a multiple-baseline design, demonstrated that the child learned the target skills and generalized their use to free play activities with her peer.

Contraindications

Very disturbed and psychotic children usually object to a puppet show because it is a threat to their attempt to maintain their grip on reality (Woltman, 1940).

Applications

Puppet play has been used effectively for both assessment and therapeutic purposes with children presenting with a wide variety of presenting problems.

References

Bender, L., & Woltman, A. (1936). The use of puppet shows as a therapeutic method for problem behaviors in children. *American Journal of Orthopsychiatry*, 6, 342–354.

Bratton, B., & Ray, D. (1999). Group puppetry. In D. Sweeney & L. Homeyer (Eds.), *The handbook of group play therapy* (pp. 267–277). San Francisco: Jossey-Bass.

Bromfield, R. (1995). The use of puppets in play therapy. *Child and Adolescent Social Work Journal*, 12(6), 435–444.

Butler, S., Guterman, J., & Rudes, J. (2009). Using puppets with children in narrative therapy to externalize the problem. *Journal of Mental Health Counseling, 31*(3), 225–233.

Carter, R., & Mason, P. (1998). The selection and use of puppets in counseling. *Professional School Counseling, 1*(5), 1–13.

Cassell, S. (1965). Effect of brief puppet therapy upon emotional responses of children undergoing cardiac catheterization. *Journal of Consulting Psychology, 29*(1), 1–8.

Gil, E. (2015). *Play in family therapy* (2nd ed.). New York: Guilford Press.

Gil, E., Sobol, B., & Bailey, C. (2005). *Children in family therapy: Using the family as a resource.* New York: Norton.

Gronna, S., Serna, L., Kennedy, C., & Prater, M. (1999). Promoting generalized social interactions using puppets and script training in an integrated preschool. *Behavior Modification, 23*(3), 419–440.

Hawkey, L. (1951). The use of puppets in child psychotherapy. *British Journal of Medical Psychology, 24*, 206–214.

Irwin, E. (1993). Using puppets for assessment. In C. E. Schaefer & D. Cangelosi (Eds.), *Play therapy techniques* (pp. 69–87). Northvale, NJ: Jason Aronson.

Irwin, E., & Malloy, E. (1975). Family puppet interviews. *Family Process, 14*, 179–191.

Jenkins, R., & Beckh, E. (1942). Finger puppets and mask making as media for work with children. *American Journal of Orthopsychiatry, 12*(2), 294–300.

Measelle, J. R., Ablow, J., Cowan, P., & Cowan, C. P. (1998). Assessing young children's views of their academic, social, and emotional lives: An evaluation of the self-perception scales of the Berkeley Puppet Interview. *Child Development, 69*(6), 1556–1576.

Narcavage, C. (1997). Using a puppet to create a symbolic client. In H. G. Kaduson & C. E. Schaefer (Eds.), *101 favorite play therapy techniques* (pp. 199–203). Northvale, NJ: Jason Aronson.

Pedro-Carroll, J., & Jones, S. (2005). A preventive play intervention to foster children's resilience in the aftermath of divorce. In L. Reddy, T. Files-Hall, & C. E. Schaefer (Eds.), *Empirically based play interventions for children* (pp. 51–75). Washington, DC: American Psychological Association.

Shapiro, D. (1995). Puppet modeling technique for children undergoing stressful medical procedures: Tips for clinicians. *International Journal of Play Therapy, 4*(2), 31–40.

Waelder, A. C. (1933). The psychoanalytic theory of play. *Psychoanalytic Quarterly, 2*, 208–224.

Wittenborn, A., Faber, A., Harvey, A., & Thomas, V. (2006). Emotionally focused family therapy and play therapy techniques. *American Journal of Family Therapy, 34*, 333–342.

Woltman, A. C. (1940). The use of puppets in understanding children. *Mental Hygiene, 24*(1), 445–458.

Part Four

CREATIVE ARTS TECHNIQUES

24

Color Your Life

Art is but one form of play.
—HERBERT SPENCER

Introduction

Kevin O'Connor (1983) developed the color-your-life technique in his work with a group of pediatric inpatients with chronic asthma. The goals of this engaging activity are to teach children about various feeling states, to facilitate the expression of their feelings, and to connect their feelings to specific events they have experienced in their lives. It is critical for children in therapy to develop skills for managing their affect and to express their feelings in an appropriate manner.

Rationale

This technique helps school-age children become aware of and express their personal feelings, which are often difficult for them to express in words. It also aids them in moving from acting out their feelings to a more adaptive form of verbal expression (Raynor & Manderino, 1989). The use of drawings, toys, and other props to aid children to identify and express their emotions has become a very popular technique in the field of play therapy. Among the numerous variations of this emotion-focused technique are "bag of feelings"; "feelings bingo"; "feelings charades"; "feelings charts"; "feelings faces"; and the "feelings word game."

Description

Ages

Six to 12 years.

115

Materials

A box of crayons and a sheet of white paper (8½ × 11 inches).

Techniques

First, the therapist asks the child to color code common feelings by pairing four to eight feelings with specific crayon colors (e.g., blue with sad, red with angry, yellow with happy, black with scared, green with jealous, orange with excited, purple with rage, and gray with lonesome). These are the colors that research indicates that children most frequently associate with these feelings (Ammen, Semrad, Soria, Limberg, & Peterson, 1996). In a variation of the technique, the child can be asked to create a personalized color code.

The child is then given a blank sheet of paper given the following instruction:

> Pretend this paper shows your whole life, from the time you were born until now. Use the crayons to color in all the feelings you have had your entire life. If you have been happy about half the time in your life then half the paper should be yellow. If you have been happy your whole life with no other feelings then you should color the whole paper yellow. You may fill the paper any way you like. (O'Connor, 1983, p. 253)

The child may complete the drawing in whatever way he/she chooses, such as using squares, circles, designs, a pie chart, and so forth. Once the child has completed the drawing, the therapist asks clarifying questions, such as "I wonder if you are feeling this way now?"; "What happens when you feel lonely?"; and "Tell me about a time you felt really scared." If the technique is used with a group, the children will often naturally compare drawings, and a lively conversation will ensue.

Variations

Therapists have structured the task by preparing different shapes for the child to color in, such as a large circle, a heart, a gingerbread man, and a child's body (to color in areas where specific feelings are felt—e.g., anger). They have also varied the drawing instruction by suggesting the child color his/her feelings related to a particular time, place, or person—for example:

"Color your current life."
"Color your house."
"Color your family."
"Color your school life."
"Color your feelings since your father died."
"Color your feelings toward your brother."
"Color your feelings for the week."

The child is asked to remember the feelings he/she had during the past week and color in the amount of each feeling. This activity is often used on an ongoing basis to monitor progress or lack thereof—for example, in the "feelings chart" technique (Bongiovani, 2003), the therapist gives the child a sheet of paper that is divided into eight vertical columns with a feeling such as happy, sad, angry, scared, proud, lonely, and so on written at the bottom of each column. The child then chooses a color to represent each feeling. Finally, the child decides how much of each feeling he/she is experiencing and colors in each column accordingly. The therapist and child then discuss factors that may be causing the feelings.

Empirical Findings

In a study of 5- and 6-year-old children's emotional association to colors, Boyatzis and Varghase (1994) found that they had positive reactions to bright colors (pink, blue, red) and negative reactions to dark colors (brown, black, gray). Girls in particular showed a preference for bright colors and a dislike for darker colors.

Applications

Color your life is widely used with children exhibiting diverse presenting problems. The basic requirement is that the children are able to recognize and name colors as well as various affective states. The technique is especially useful for children who are not very verbal and can express their feelings better through drawings. The writers have used it successfully with preschool children ages 4–6 years who are able to recognize the four basic emotions of mad, glad, sad, and scared. The technique can be used in an individual or group format. As a monitoring tool, it is helpful to use the technique at several points throughout the therapy in order to observe what affective changes have occurred.

References

Ammen, S., Semrad, J., Soria, S., Limberg, E., & Peterson, C. (1996). The development of tools to research the color-your-life technique. *International Journal of Play Therapy*, 5(2), 21–39.

Bongiovani, M. (2003). The feelings chart. In H. G. Kaduson & C. E. Schaefer (Eds.), *101 favorite play therapy techniques* (Vol. 3, pp. 84–87). Northvale, NJ: Jason Aronson.

Boyatzis, C., & Varghase, R. (1994). Children's emotional associations with colors. *Journal of Genetic Psychology*, 155, 77–85.

O'Connor, K. (1983). The color-your-life technique. In C. E. Schaefer & K. J. O'Connor (Eds.), *Handbook of play therapy* (pp. 251–288). New York: Wiley.

Raynor, C., & Manderino, M. (1998). "Color your life": An assessment and treatment strategy for children. *Journal of Child and Adolescent Psychiatric and Mental Health Nursing*, 2(2), 28–51.

25

Clay Play

> And man is made from the clay of the earth. . . .
> —GENESIS 1:24

Introduction

Clay, sand, dirt, and water are basic elements of the earth and have formed the basis of children's play from ancient times. Clay play refers to the process of handling, manipulating, and sculpting clay, and the products of these activities (Sholt & Gavron, 2006). Using clay in therapy taps into the most fundamental human experience: touch. You need very little skill to manipulate clay or play dough and there is hardly any chance of failure. Although children have always played with clay, more recently it has become a valuable technique for play therapists because children are naturally motivated to engage in clay play (Moustakas, 1953).

The term *play dough* refers to the many natural and man-made clays and doughs. For therapeutic use with younger children, we recommend the commercial Play-Doh brand because it offers children product familiarity and consistency, as well as easy manipulation and clean up.

Rationale

The healing powers of clay play include:

- *Sensory pleasure.* Children derive tactile, kinesthetic, and visual pleasure from handling clay, which contributes to their overall sense of well-being.

- *Verbal self-expression.* Often clay play enables children to express deep issues, as the sensory experience seems to loosen their tongue. When children have soothing, comforting things to hold with their hands, talking about difficult things can become easier (Oaklander, 1988). There are many accounts in the literature describing how the creation of clay figures lead to the expression of powerful emotions that previously were inaccessible to the client (Henly, 2002; Sholt & Gavron, 2006). In addition to conscious self-expression, the primitive nature of clay can help bring repressed ideas, feelings, impulses, and memories into conscious awareness (Betensky, 1995).

• *Ego boosting.* Clay play tends to enhance children's sense of competence and control because it is easy to roll it into balls and snakes. In real life, many children have little or no control over what is happening in their world.

• *Relaxation.* Touching and manipulating clay or play dough is a soothing, calming experience for children.

• *Catharsis.* Pounding clay is a simple but effective way for children to express and release angry feelings in a nonverbal way—for example, smashing, tearing, stabbing, throwing the clay.

• *Positive affect.* Playing with clay can elevate one's mood when feeling anxious, bored, or sad.

• *Concretization.* Concretization refers to the process in which inner thoughts, feelings, fantasies, and conflicts are embodied in concrete, external objects and thus made more understandable to children (Sholt & Gavron, 2006).

• *Revealing unconscious material.* Clay work can evoke the direct expression of unconscious material that is not filtered through the client's mind (Anderson, 1955). The primitive nature of clay can bring repressed ideas, feelings, and memories into conscious awareness (Betensky, 1995; Winship & Haigh, 1998).

Description

Ages

Three years and up.

Materials

The materials needed for this type of play include cans of easy-to-use play dough and a few simple tools such as a pencil to poke holes in the clay, and a popsicle stick to cut the clay. Also, a smooth surface, a vinyl mat to work the clay on, and a moist cloth or sponge to clean your hands make for ease of use.

Children ages 6–12 years tend to prefer regular, self-hardening clay to play dough. This modeling clay is great for making different shapes and objects, such as animals and human figures, but it takes extra effort to soften and be workable.

Techniques

Free Clay Play

In this nondirective approach, children ages 3 years and up are provided with a flat tray and given free rein to use a piece of play dough (baseball size or larger) or clay to make anything he/she wishes (e.g., roll it into tubes, ball it up, pound it into a pancake, or create a figure out of it). Sometimes the spontaneous play with clay is purely sensory (e.g., squeezing and molding). This pleasurable sensory experience often makes the expression of troublesome thoughts and emotions easier (this is true with clients of any age, including teens and adults).

If the child is reluctant to use the clay, the therapist may model the enthusiastic use of it—for example, by making the child's favorite animal. More often, the therapist gives the child specific directions on how to use the play dough or clay, including the following structured techniques:

Cathartic Clay Play

Play dough and clay are excellent materials for helping children express their anger. This can be done with a ball of play dough/clay or the child can make a person or monster out of it first. The therapist simply asks the child to pound or smash the play dough with his/her fist. It is a safe way to release anger. One way to do this technique is to ask the child to think of something he/she gets angry about before smashing the play dough. The therapist then takes a turn and does likewise (e.g., "I get angry when I see someone being bullied"). Finally, the therapist discusses with the child the difference between hitting the play dough and hitting other people.

Stress Relief Clay Play

The manipulation of a piece of play dough or clay can serve as an effective relaxant similar to that of a stress ball or fidget toy. In this regard, a number of university professors hand out containers of play dough to help students quickly relax and focus attention during the most stressful weeks of the semester.

Self-Figure

The child is asked to create him/herself out of play dough—a variation of the draw-a-family technique in Chapter 33. The goal is for the therapist to gain insight into the self-concept of the child by observing if the self-figure looks capable, friendly, happy, tiny, and so forth.

Group Clay Play

First, give each child in the peer group a fair-size piece of play dough (at least a baseball size) and a flat work surface. Tell the group that you will begin something with your clay and then each group member will get a chance to add to the initial shape with their play dough. Urge them to create whatever they wish while assuring them that it does not have to be real or representational. The only requirement is to add something to the original shape. You then mold something rather nondescript from your clay and hand it to one of the group members next to you. Each child adds something to the construction and passes it on to one of the children sitting next to him/her. Keep the tone of the activity light and fun and be sure that it moves quickly to keep the group's interest. A group discussion follows the completion of the task. The goal is to foster cooperation, communication, bonding, and positive affect in the group members.

Family Clay Play

A family is asked to jointly use the play dough to create characters and then tell a story about them. The goal is for the therapist to gain insight about feelings, concerns, and interactions of family members.

Clay Metaphors

The child is asked to create a three-dimensional object out of play dough to represent a troublesome feeling, thought, or behavior (e.g., something that makes you afraid or happy). Or the child might be asked to make a figure representing him/herself or his/her mother. In regard to the latter, a child might respond to this by making a snake or angel figure representing his/her mother. Alternately, a child might be asked to make a play dough figure that represents and externalizes a personal, troublesome behavior, such as encopresis.

Clay Play Coaching

Elementary school children can be taught how to make clay objects such as dogs and dinosaurs—for example, they might be taught how to poke a hole in a ball of play dough using a pencil and then insert a clay arm or leg in the hole and pinch it closed with their thumb and forefinger. To make a pinch pot, you use your thumbs to push a hole in a ball of clay, and then form rudimentary walls for the pot by pinching the clay and turning the pot. The clay pot is then pushed on a flat surface to create a base (White, 2006). The creation of these simple objects can boost a child's ego and self-confidence.

Empirical Findings

1. A survey by Sholt and Gavron (2006) found that 99% of play therapists believed that clay play was therapeutic, but only 25% of them reported that they use it in their practice. Clearly, there is a need to expand its inclusion in the play therapy toolbox of clinicians.

2. Feldman, Villanueva, and Devroede (1993) used modeling clay as a metaphor for feces with six school-age children experiencing refractory encopresis. The clay play in which the children expressed their feelings of disgust and aggression resulted in significant improvement in four of the six children.

3. In a randomly controlled trial with college students, Kimport and Robbins (2012) found that manipulating clay for 5 minutes resulted in a greater reduction in the students' negative mood than did squeezing a stress ball for 5 minutes. Structured clay play—for example, making a pinch pot—resulted in greater reduction in the negative mood of the students than did free clay play.

4. Rahman and Moheb (2010) found that clay play by 6-year-old children resulted in a significant reduction in their anxiety.

5. In a randomized, controlled trial, Bell and Robbins (2007) found that the simple act of creating a work of art, such as a clay figure, produced dramatic reductions in the negative mood and anxiety of young adults.

Applications

Clay play has been widely used to facilitate children's conscious and unconscious self-expression, as well as to overcome children's tension, anxiety, and negative moods.

References

Anderson, F. E. (1955). Catharsis and empowerment through group claywork with incest survivors. *Arts in Psychotherapy, 22*(5), 413–427.

Bell, C., & Robbins, S. (2007). Effect of art production on negative mood: A randomized, controlled trial. *Art Therapy: Journal of the American Art Therapy Association, 24*(2), 71–75.

Betensky, M. (1995). *What do you see?: Phenomenology of therapeutic art expression.* London: Jessica Kingsley.

Feldman, P., Villanueva, S., & Devroede, G. (1993). Use of play with clay to treat children with intractable encopresis. *Journal of Pediatrics, 122*(3), 483–488.

Henley, D. (2002). *Claywork in art therapy.* London: Jessica Kingsley.

Kimport, E., & Robbins, S. (2012). Efficacy of creative clay work for reducing negative mood: A randomized controlled trial. *Art Therapy: Journal of the American Art Therapy Association, 29*(2), 74–79.

Moustakas, C. (1953). *Children in play therapy.* New York: McGraw-Hill.

Oaklander, V. (1988). *Windows to our children: A Gestalt therapy approach to children and adolescents.* Gouldsbora, ME: Gestalt Journal Press.

Rahman, P., & Moheb, N. (2010). The effectiveness of clay therapy and narrative therapy on anxiety of pre-school children: A comparative study. *Procedia Social and Behavioral Sciences, 5*, 23–27.

Sholt, M., & Gavron, T. (2006). Therapeutic qualities of clay-work in art therapy and psychotherapy: A review. *Art Therapy: Journal of the American Art Therapy Association, 23*(2), 66–72.

White, P. R. (2006). CLAYtherapy: The clinical application of clay with children. In C. E. Schaefer & H. G. Kaduson (Eds.), *Contemporary play therapy: Theory, research, and practice* (pp. 270–292). New York: Guilford Press.

Winship, G., & Haigh, R. (1998). The formation of objects in the group matrix: Reflections on creative therapy with clay. *Group Analysis, 31*(1), 71–81.

26

Free Drawings

Every child is an artist. The problem is how to remain an artist once he grows up.

—PABLO PICASSO

Introduction

Children's drawings are visual representations made with crayons, markers, or pencils that they find nonthreatening and enjoyable. Drawings, often referred to as the universal language of childhood (Rubin, 1984), enable children to express themselves naturally and spontaneously. For decades therapists have used them to assess a child's intellectual and emotional development and for therapeutic purposes (Golomb, 1992). Up to age 7 years, children rarely decline to participate in a drawing activity.

Rationale

The therapeutic benefits of drawings by children include:

• *Therapeutic alliance.* Free drawings provide a means for the therapist to establish a rapid, easy, and pleasant rapport with a child.

• *Positive emotion.* Free drawings give children an experience of enjoyment and accomplishment.

• *Self-expression.* Free drawings are an excellent medium for children with a limited vocabulary or language difficulties to express themselves.

• *Understanding.* Free drawings are a great way for the therapist to gain better understanding of the child's inner world and struggles. Through the act of drawing children can safely project their inner thoughts and feelings about themselves and their family, as well as about their current and past experiences and difficulties.

  • *Emotional expression and verbal communication.* The act of drawing in front of a therapist seems to aid emotional expression and verbal communication and result in improved self-concept (Allan, 1978).

  • *Expression of unconscious disturbances.* Spontaneous drawings can often express unconscious disturbances because pictured projections tend to escape censorship more easily than do verbal expressions.

  • *Mastery.* By graphically representing their inner thoughts and feelings, children bring them out in the open so they are better able to confront them and learn to gain control over them.

Description

Ages

Three to 12 years.

Material

White paper and a pencil, crayon, or felt pen.

Techniques

The choice of subject matter in a free drawing is left completely up to the child. In this simple, nondirective, time-honored technique, children are given plain paper and a drawing instrument and asked to draw something, anything they wish. During the drawing process, the therapist does not make comments, ask questions, or otherwise interrupt or disturb the child. When the drawing is finished, the therapist asks open-ended questions to encourage the child to explain the picture (e.g., "Tell me about your drawing"). Alternately, the therapist may ask the child to make up a story about the drawing. A child's spontaneous drawing is a projective technique that often provides the therapist with important information about the child's inner thoughts, feelings, conflicts, and hopes. According to Oaklander (1978): "The very act of drawing, with no therapist intervention whatsoever is a powerful expression of self that helps establish one's self-identity and provides a way of expressing feelings" (p. 53).

Variations

Serial Drawing

For each session over a 6- to 10-week period, the therapist simply asks the child to draw any picture the child wishes. (See Chapter 29, "Serial Drawings.")

Crayon Drawing

Historically, ancient peoples marked up their stones using some combination of beeswax or charcoal and pigment, but these crayons were not convenient or easy to use. So teachers in the 19th century gave children slate boards and pencils made of slate or chalk to draw and write. Crayons, as we know them today, are an early 20th-century creation specifically designed to be safe, inexpensive, and colorful markers for children. The first box of crayons became available in 1903. Each box sold for a nickel and contained eight crayons of different colors. Crayons are typically the first drawing instruments tried by children. At about age 3 years children are able to make crayon drawings that represent real objects and things. Crayon drawings can be used to foster the expression of emotions by young children.

The choice of crayon colors by children ages 6–12 years often reflects their emotional state. In particular, the frequent choice of black or red colors in a child's picture could be a red flag for the therapist. Black can be an indicator of depression or feeling hopeless. Red may reflect feelings of anger. Researchers have found that children who suffered recent traumas, such as earthquakes, tend to choose more red and black colors in their drawings than other children (Cotton, 1985; Gregorian, Azarian, DeMaria, & McDonald, 1996). On the other hand, blue and green colors are usually calm ones, while yellow and orange are often selected to express cheerfulness.

Kinetic Family Drawing

An alternative to a free drawing is to structure the task by asking the child to draw his/her family doing something together. (See Chapter 33, "Draw a Family.")

Solution Drawing

Another directive drawing technique is called solution drawing. In the 1955 book *Harold and the Purple Crayon* by Crockett Johnson, a little 4-year-old boy literally colors his world by using a purple crayon to draw whatever he happens to need. In the story, when Harold finds himself in difficulty he draws his way out of the dilemma. The book illustrates the power of one's creative imagination to solve problems.

Accordingly, children ages 5 years and up can be helped to develop their problem-solving ability by first reading *Harold and the Purple Crayon* and then using a purple crayon to draw a solution to a series of fantastic problems that you present to them (e.g., "You see a huge brown bear strolling down the street and he's coming toward you. Draw a way to solve this problem" or "Draw a way to overcome times you are bored").

Solution drawings are designed to help children who have difficulty generating solutions to their problems, particularly children with "problem-solving deficit disorder" (Levin, 2007).

Self-Portrait

The child is asked to make a self-portrait using pencils, crayons, or felt pens (Berryman, 1959). The therapist directs the child by saying, "Draw a picture of yourself and try to include your whole body." This technique can be helpful in revealing hidden aspects of the child's self-concept.

Bad Dream Drawing

To aid a school-age child in overcoming a nightmare, Hunyady (1984) asked the child to draw a picture of it. He told the child: "Ancient man helped himself conquer the fear of wild animals by making drawings of them. You should therefore make a drawing of what frightened you in the dream and if you succeed, you have already conquered it." He found that children were often able to laugh at the monster they had drawn.

Draw Yourself as an Animal

The therapist asks the child to "Draw the animal you would choose to be if you could be any animal." The therapist and child later discuss the reasons the child selected that animal.

Scribble Drawing

Ask the child to close his/her eyes and scribble all over a piece of paper with a pencil. Once complete, ask the child to look at the scribble drawing and try to see recognizable objects in the scribble. The premise is that the children will project aspects from their unconscious by this method.

Empirical Findings

1. Based on a meta-analysis, Driessnack (2005) reports that the opportunity to draw while talking increases the amount of verbal information children report during a clinical interview.

2. Woolford, Patterson, Macleod, Hobbs, and Hayne (2015) found that school-age children who were asked to draw and tell about their presenting problem provided twice as much verbal information as children asked to tell only.

3. Both Patterson and Hayne (2011) and Wesson and Salmon (2001) reported that children ages 5–12 years who were asked to draw and tell about emotional events they had experienced reported more information than children asked to tell only.

4. Gross and Hayne (1998) found that children ages 3–6 years who were given the opportunity to draw and tell about their emotional experiences reported more than twice as much information than children asked to tell only.

Applications

Drawing activities can be used with most children to facilitate conscious and unconscious self-expression. Drawing techniques are particularly appropriate for children who are shy; anxious; have speech and language difficulties, such as selective mutism; or speak a different language than the therapist.

References

Allan, J. (1978). Serial drawing: A therapeutic approach with young children. *Canadian Counsellor, 12*, 223–228.

Berryman, E. (1959). The self-portrait: A suggested extension of the H.T.P. *Perceptual and Motor Skills, 9*, 411–414.

Cotton, M. (1985). Creative art expression from a leukemic child. *Art Therapy, 2*, 55–65.

Driessnack, M. (2005). Children's drawings as facilitators of communication: A meta-analysis. *Journal of Pediatric Nursing, 20*(6), 415–423.

Golomb, C. (1992). *The child's creation of a pictorial world.* Berkeley: University of California Press.

Gregorian, V., Azarian, A., DeMaria, M., & McDonald, L. (1996). Color of disaster: The psychology of the "black sun." *Arts in Psychotherapy, 23*, 1–14.

Gross, J., & Hayne, H. (1998). Drawing facilitates children's verbal reports of emotionally laden events. *Journal of Experimental Psychology: Applied, 4*(2), 163–179.

Hunyady, H. (1984). A report on a drawing therapy for children's nightmares. *Journal of Evolutionary Psychology, 5*, 129–130.

Johnson, C. (1955). *Harold and the purple crayon.* New York: HarperCollins.

Levin, D. (2007). Problem solving deficit disorder. In E. Goodenough (Ed.), *Where do the children play?* (pp. 264–285). Detroit: Michigan Television.

Oaklander, V. (1978). *Windows to our children.* Moab, VT: Real People Press.

Patterson, T., & Hayne, H. (2011). Does drawing facilitate older children's reports of emotionally laden events? *Applied Cognitive Psychology, 25*(1), 119–126.

Rubin, J. (1984). *Child art therapy: Understanding and helping children grow through art* (2nd ed.). New York: Van Nostrand Reinhold.

Wesson, M., & Salmon, K. (2001). Drawing and showing: Helping children to report emotionally laden events. *Applied Cognitive Psychology, 15*, 302–320.

Woolford, J., Patterson, T., Macleod, E., Hobbs, L., & Hayne, H. (2015). Drawing helps children to talk about their presenting problem during a mental health assessment. *Clinical Child Psychology and Psychiatry, 20*(1), 68–83.

27

Trauma Drawings

Introduction

Drawing is a natural and enjoyable mode of communication by children. It offers a way to express thoughts and feelings in a manner that is less threatening than verbal means alone. Pynoos and Eth (1986) observed that drawings were used as early as the First World War to help individuals access repressed memories of traumatic scenes. Counselors and psychotherapists have often asked children to draw traumatic events because they generally lack the communication skills to explain what they have witnessed or directly experienced. Also, children are likely to feel psychological distance from the event by drawing it, as if they were discussing an event in a book or on television.

Rationale

The expression and disclosure of previously experienced traumatic events has been found to be associated with better physical and mental health (Smyth & Helm, 2003). For a child who has experienced a single-incident trauma, drawing the traumatic event can help the child to express thoughts and feelings too painful to speak about directly. For many years, it was believed that children should not be asked to talk about these traumatic memories for fear of retraumatizing the child. However, it is now known that it is important to the healing process to provide children with ways to express their fears and worries and to provide sensory experiences that facilitate access to their feelings.

Trauma memories are stored in both hemispheres of the brain but primarily in the right hemisphere. Rational thinking, words, and logic are hindered by trauma. Thus, the most effective therapy focuses on activating the trauma memories of the child through nonverbal right-brain activity, such as drawing or play

129

reenactments. Then the child will be better able to make sense of and assimilate the experience through language and logical analysis (left-brain functions). So it is best if both sides of the brain work together to process and mentally digest the trauma incident.

The idea that trauma is encoded primarily in a sensory manner by the mind and body is now widely accepted by professionals who work with clients exhibiting traumatic stress reactions. According to van der Kolk (1994), the trauma memory needs to be initially processed through a sensory memory, such as a drawing, so that it can be transformed into a verbal narrative. He believes that then and only then can the person tell the story of what happened. Drawing assists in reducing the anxious reactivity of a child to trauma memories through repeated visual reexposure in a medium that is perceived and felt by the child to be safe (Malchiodi, 1998).

Description

Ages

Three to 12 years.

Technique

Draw and Tell about the Trauma

When a child experiences a trauma, drawing "what happened" has been found very therapeutic. Pynoos and Eth (1986) discovered that, in order to successfully resolve and master a traumatic event, children need the opportunity to re-create the experience in detail. To facilitate the healing process of a child after a trauma, they described a structured interview that includes asking the child to draw the trauma. While it is a difficult task to re-create an image on paper of the traumatic event, most children find some relief in finally being asked to describe what happened.

In the initial session with a recently traumatized child, Pynoos and Eth (1986) recommend that the therapist help school-age children express the personal impact of the trauma through a projective free drawing and subsequently telling a story about the drawing. The motor (drawing) and the verbal (tell a story about it) actions help move the child from a passive, powerless involvement with the trauma to a feeling of active control over the experience. First, the child is given a pencil and blank piece of paper (8½ × 11 inches) and asked to "Draw whatever you like but something you can tell a story about." Then the therapist encourages the child to elaborate further on both the drawing and the story (e.g., "What happens next?"). The key premise of a free drawing is that the trauma event remains intrusive on the child's mind and will likely be projected somewhere in the drawing or story. The therapist's task is to identify the trauma reference, which may be obvious or subtle.

The next step is for the therapist to link some aspect of the drawing and storytelling to the trauma event (e.g., "I bet you wish your father was still here to protect you"). The third step is to encourage the child to re-create the event (e.g., "Now is a good time to tell what happened and what you saw"). The child may first choose to reexperience the trauma in drawings or play enactments but the therapist must assist the child to translate the play action or pictorial depiction into words that describe the sensory experience (e.g., "Boy, you must have gotten blood all over you!"). The role of the therapist during this process is to provide a safe and protected environment so the child can work on mastering the trauma experience. The final step is provide closure by reviewing and summarizing the session, and to reassure the child that it is all right to have felt helpless and afraid at the time of the event and then sad or angry afterward.

Variation

Emotional Mastery (Shelby, 1997; Shelby & Tredinick, 1995)

First, children ages 3–8 years are encouraged to draw a picture of what happened during the traumatic event (e.g., earthquake, hurricane, dog attack). Second, they are asked to express their feelings toward their drawing (e.g., "I don't like you because you scared me!"). Third, they are instructed to do whatever they wish to the drawing to express their negative feelings and gain a sense of mastery over it (e.g., tearing up the picture, scribbling all over it, or crumbling it into a ball and throwing it against a wall).

Empirical Findings

1. Gross and Haynes (1998) conducted a series of studies to explore how and if drawing facilitated verbal reports in children ages 3–6 years. The results supported the premise that drawing does indeed appear to enhance children's communication of feelings and perceptions. In their initial investigation they compared two groups of children: one group that talked about their experience while they drew, and a second group that were simply asked to tell about their experiences. The children who were given the opportunity to draw while talking about their experiences did report more information than the children who were merely asked to talk. A second experiment was conducted (Patterson & Hayne, 2009) to examine older children, ages 5–12 years, who were interviewed with both procedures. It also revealed that children do report two or three times more information when asked to draw and tell about an emotionally laden event. According to the authors, drawing seemed to help memory retrieval because trauma and drawing are largely sensory experiences.

2. In support of earlier findings by Hayne and colleagues, Woolford (2011) found that school-age children who were asked to draw and tell about their presenting problem provided twice as much information as children who told only. Also, the meta-analytic study by Driessnack (2005) discovered that giving children the opportunity to draw during a clinical interview resulted in significantly more information by the children than just a verbal interview. This strategy resulted in a large overall effect size of 0.95.

Applications

Since drawing is a modality that addresses the sensory experiences inherent in trauma, it is an effective tool for debriefing, resolution, and healing for childhood victims of trauma.

References

Driessnack, M. (2005). Children's drawings as facilitators of communication: A meta-analysis. *Journal of Pediatric Nursing, 20*(6), 415–423.

Gross, J., & Haynes, H. (1998). Drawing facilitates children's verbal reports of emotionally laden events. *Journal of Experimental Psychology, 4,* 163–179.

Malchiodi, C. A. (1998). *Understanding children's drawings.* New York: Guilford Press.

Patterson, T., & Hayne, H. (2009). Does drawing facilitate older children's reports of emotionally laden events? *Applied Cognitive Psychology, 25*(1), 119–126.

Pynoos, R., & Eth, S. (1986). Witness to violence: The Child Interview. *Journal of the American Academy of Child Psychiatry, 25*(3), 306–319.

Shelby, J. (1997). Rubble, disruption, and tears: Helping young survivors of natural disaster. In H. G. Kaduson, D. Cangelosi, & C. Schaefer (Eds.), *The playing cure* (pp. 143–169). Northvale, NJ: Jason Aronson.

Shelby, J., & Tredinick, M (1995). Crisis intervention with survivors of natural disaster: Lessons from Hurricane Andrew. *Journal of Counseling and Development, 73*(5), 491–497.

Smyth, J., & Helm, R. (2003). Focused expressive writing as self-help for stress and trauma. *Journal of Clinical Psychology, 59,* 227–235.

Van der Kolk, S. (1994). The body keeps the score: Memory and the evolving psychobiology of posttraumatic stress. *Harvard Review of Psychiatry, 1*(5), 253–265.

Woolford, J. (2010). *Clinical assessment of the child: Does drawing help children talk about their presenting problems?* Master's thesis, University of Otago, New Zealand.

28

Mandala Drawings

I knew that in finding the mandala as an expression of the self I had attained what was for me the ultimate. Perhaps someone else knows more, but not I.

—CARL G. JUNG

Introduction

The mandala, which means "circle" in Sanskrit, has a long history and is known for its spiritual significance among many cultures. The traditional shape of most mandalas is a square with four gates containing a circle with a center point. However, many mandalas are simple circles that do not include the outer square. Mandalas often signify balance. In religious practices, they are used as symbols and tools for meditation, protection, and healing. They are often present in the sacred art of both Hindu and Buddhist traditions but have also been found in cave drawings, sand paintings, and Gothic rose windows.

In Tibetan Buddhism, the creation of sand mandalas is a sacred meditative ritual. Monks carefully arrange colored sand to reproduce intricate symbols. This painstaking process can take days or even weeks. When the "mandala of colored powders" is completed, a closing ceremony takes place and the sand mandala is destroyed. The sand is swept up and handfuls are given to those who participated in the ceremony as a symbol of possibility. The rest of the sand is thrown into a body of water to spread its spiritual energy and bless the world. The underlying message of the mandala ceremony is that nothing is permanent—a pivotal Buddhist teaching (Chittister, 2011).

Navajo Indians create sand mandalas as part of their healing ceremonies. Their mandalas are also created with precision and include images of Yei, Navajo spirits, who are called upon to heal and restore harmony. Similarly, medicine wheels, or sacred hoops, have been used for healing by generations of various

Native American tribes. The medicine wheel can be a piece of artwork or a physical construction on the land.

Forms that are similar to mandalas are common in Christianity as well. These include the Celtic cross that combines a cross with a ring surrounding the intersection, rose windows that are circular and often found in Gothic-style architecture, and the rosary cross. Many people have also noted that the pattern of a mandala (a circle with a center) is found in biology (e.g., form of cells), botany (form of flowers), and chemistry (form of atoms).

Giordano Bruno, an Italian living during the Renaissance, introduced the idea of using the mandala as a therapeutic tool. He believed that using visualization exercises and memorizing mandala images would result in a personal transformation and bring about harmony and positive changes.

Mandalas were first used in therapy by Carl Jung (1973, 1989). Jung (1989) painted and drew mandalas as part of his personal analysis and found that they corresponded to his internal experiences and psychic transformations from day to day. He found that the act of drawing mandalas not only had a calming effect but also was a symbol of self-striving toward integration, wholeness, and individuation. Jung wrote:

> When I began drawing the mandalas, I saw that everything, all paths I had been following, all the steps I had taken, were leading back to a single point—namely, to the mid-point. It became increasingly plain to me that the mandala is the center. It is the exponent of all paths. It is the path to the center, to individuation. (p. 196)

Rationale

Mandalas are symbolic tools for gaining insight and understanding. They have a wide variety of therapeutic benefits.

- *Communication.* Mandalas provide a way for children to draw subconscious images, metaphors, and symbols that provide valuable information about their personalities and internal struggles. The shapes and colors created often reflect internal experiences and emotions and can be used to access unconscious material.

- *Insight.* Completed mandalas can be seen as representations or snapshots of the creator's psyche or internal world. Jungian play therapists do not analyze children's mandalas. Instead, they help children interpret and find meaning from their own internal experience.

- *Psychic healing.* Jung believed that the circular image of the mandala helps individuals to synthesize information and experiences when confusing or disorienting situations occur. He wrote:

The severe pattern imposed by the circular image of this kind compensates the disorder and confusion of the psychic state—namely through the construction of a central point to which everything is related, or by a concentric arrangement of the disordered multiplicity and the contradictory and irreconcilable elements. (1983, p. 236)

• *Relaxation.* Research has shown that making or coloring mandalas shifts the brain into a meditative/alpha wave state characterized by a sense of calm and relaxation (Beaucaire, 2012; Green, 2013).

• *Attention and self-regulation.* Green (2013) noted that creating mandalas is a cognitive and intention-based process characterized by self-regulation and attention to the present.

• *Access to unconscious material.* The projective nature of mandalas makes them a powerful tool for understanding the internal world of children.

• *Concretization.* Mandalas provide a concrete picture of the child's psyche and his/her attempts at achieving a sense of balance and resolution.

• *Enjoyment.* Creating, coloring, and painting mandalas is an enjoyable, fulfilling process. In addition, the integrative, healing qualities of the finished mandala brings about a sense of well-being.

Description

Ages

Four years and up.

Materials

Because the coloring of mandalas by children should not be very complicated, present them with a box of crayons and a sheet of white paper containing a circular mandala design. The mandala should contain simple shapes that children can color in, such as hearts and flowers. Some children may prefer simple abstract shapes. Alternately, give a child a sheet of paper with a large circle drawn on it and ask the child to draw and color in whatever he/she wishes.

Free, printable mandala templates ranging from simple to very complex are available on the Internet (e.g., *www.mandala-4free.de/en/index.htm*). Also, a number of mandala coloring books and games are available for young children—for example, *My First Mandalas Coloring Book* (Pomaska, 2008), and *Kids' First Mandalas* (Verlag, 2005) include child-friendly images such as hearts, circles, flowers, and insects. Mandala kits such as the Mandala Designer (ages 6 years and up) and the Junior Mandala Designer (ages 4 years and up) include stencils, colored pens, and a drawing station.

Techniques

Mandalas are helpful for any child who is able to color. Depending on the child's artistic skill and stage of development, mandalas can be created from scratch or, more commonly, predrawn mandalas can be used. Jungian play therapists often recommend using predrawn mandalas with children before asking them to create their own. This provides a concrete experience with the medium, which is especially important for young children (Green, Drewes, & Kominski, 2013).

Mandalas are often introduced with a guided imagery exercise designed to encourage relaxation and creativity. However, this is not required and most therapists prefer to simply ask children to color a predrawn mandala without an opening exercise.

Variation

Trauma Mandala

Henderson, Rosen, and Mascaro (2007) asked college undergraduates suffering from posttraumatic stress disorder (PTSD) to draw a large circle on a piece of paper and then fill the circle with representations of feelings or emotions related to their trauma using symbols, designs, and colors (but no words) that felt right to them. Compared with a control group, the participants in the experimental group reported greater decreases in symptoms of trauma at a 1-month follow-up.

Empirical Findings

1. Curry and Kasser (2005) examined the effectiveness of different types of coloring activities for reducing anxiety. Eighty-four undergraduate students experienced a brief anxiety induction and were randomly assigned to color a mandala, plaid design, or a blank piece of paper. Results of this experiment showed that anxiety levels decreased in the mandala and plaid coloring groups to a greater extent than in the control group. These findings show that coloring of a complex geometric pattern may induce a relaxed state that benefits individuals suffering from anxiety. Coloring therapy combines aspects of art therapy (i.e., coloring a form) and meditation (i.e., deeply concentrating on an experience that is soothing).

2. Van der Vennet and Serice (2012) replicated the Curry and Kasser (2005) study using the State Anxiety Inventory after an anxiety-inducing writing activity, and again after coloring either a mandala design, a plaid design, or a blank paper. In this experiment, coloring a mandala reduced anxiety to a significantly greater degree than coloring on a plaid design or blank paper.

3. Green and colleagues (2013) described the use of mandalas with adolescents diagnosed with ADHD. Analysis of one of the participants demonstrated that coloring mandalas decreased the boy's stress, helped him communicate about his internal and external struggles and increased his awareness of his personal strength. Also noteworthy is the finding by Smitheman-Brown and Church (1996) that mandala drawing increased concentration abilities and decreased impulsive behavior in children ages 10–13 years diagnosed with ADD or ADHD.

Applications

Mandalas can be used with children, adolescents, and adults. They are an excellent tool for relaxation, stress management, self-regulation, and self-reflection. Mandala coloring is especially useful for treating anxiety-related disorders, PTSD, ADHD, and individuals who can benefit from self-reflection and insight-oriented therapy.

References

Beaucare, M. (2012). *The art of mandala meditation.* Avon, MA: Adams Media.

Chittister, J. (2011, November 20). The mandala: Why do monks destroy it? Retrieved from *www.huffingtonpost.com/sister-joan-chittister-osb/mandala-why-destroy-it_b_970479. html.*

Curry, N. A., & Kasser, T. (2005). Can coloring mandalas reduce anxiety? *Art Therapy: Journal of the American Art Therapy Association, 22,* 81–85.

Green, E. J. (2013*). Mandalas and meaning: A coloring workbook for adolescents.* Dallas, TX: Author.

Green, E. J., Drewes, A. A., & Kominski, J. M. (2013). Use of mandalas in Jungian play therapy with adolescents diagnosed with ADHD. *International Journal of Play Therapy, 22*(3), 159–172.

Jung, C. (1973). *Mandala symbolism* (R. F. C. Hull, Trans.). Princeton, NJ: Princeton University Press. (Original work published 1959)

Jung, C. G. (1983). Integration, wholeness, and the self. In A. Storr (Ed.), *The essential Jung* (pp. 227–238). Princeton, NJ: Princeton University Press.

Jung, C. G. (1989). Confrontation with the unconscious. In A. Jaffe (Ed.), *Memories, dreams, reflections* (pp. 170–199) (C. Winston & R. Winston, Trans.). New York: Vintage Books.

Pomaska, A. (2008). *My first mandalas coloring book.* Mineola, NY: Dover Coloring Books.

Smitheman-Brown, V., & Church, R. (1996). Mandala drawing: Facilitating creative growth in children with ADD or ADHD. *Art Therapy: Journal of the American Art Therapy Association, 13*(4), 252–262.

Van der Vennet, R., & Serice, S. (2012). Can coloring mandalas reduce anxiety?: A replication study. *Art Therapy: Journal of the American Art Therapy Association, 29,* 87–92.

Verlag, A. (2005). *Kids' first mandalas.* New York: Sterling.

29

Serial Drawings

Often the hands will solve a mystery that the intellect has struggled with in vain.

—Carl G. Jung

Introduction

The serial drawing technique, introduced by Jungian play therapist John Allan (1978), involves asking the child to "draw a picture" repeatedly over time. The drawings done each session include little or no direction from the therapist and the child draws anything he/she wishes. It is the *serial* nature of the activity (i.e., regular meetings) and the fact that the child shares the drawings with an understanding therapist that activates the healing process (Allan, 1988). The method is based on Jung's belief that examining dreams and works of symbolic expression as a whole, over time, provides a more comprehensive understanding of the individual's unconscious inner world. Rooted in Jung's belief in the self-healing ability of the psyche, focus is on where the unconscious leads and how it evolves. What transpires in one or two play sessions is not as significant as the form that the image, fantasy, or behavior takes over time (Allan & Levin, 1993). With the moderately disturbed child, significant therapeutic change tends to be seen in serial drawings over about 10 sessions (Allan, 1977).

The themes of serial drawings commonly go through three phases that correspond to the stages of therapy: initial, middle, and termination (Allan, 1977, 1978). During the initial phase (Sessions 1–3), drawings commonly reflect a view of the child's internal world, the effects of the child's difficulties and his/her sense of helplessness, and the vehicle for building a relationship with the therapist. During the middle phase (Sessions 4–7), drawings reflect a separation between painful feelings and other feelings, a deeper relationship to the therapist, and increased communication about the child's issues. Finally, during the termination phase

(Sessions 8–10), drawings show mastery, self-control and worth, positive imagery, humor, and removal of attachment to the therapist.

Rationale

The sequential nature of the serial drawing technique and the fact that the child shares his/her drawings with an emotionally responsive therapist provides a number of therapeutic benefits:

- *Overcoming resistance.* Drawing is a child-friendly, nonthreatening activity that decreases discomfort and resistance in children. This is especially important when children are unable or unwilling to discuss difficulties or feel forced to attend therapy. In addition, the fact that children get to choose the medium they wish to work with—such as pencils, crayons, paint, clay, or storytelling—makes serial drawings an especially enjoyable activity (Allan, 1978).

- *Communication.* Serial drawings are projective in nature because they allow children to create whatever image they desire. This provides access to important information regarding children's internal experiences, perceptions, struggles, and resources, as well as underlying unconscious processes.

- *Creative thinking.* Expression of conflicts through serial drawings promotes problem solving, innovative thinking, flexibility, and emotional growth. This process helps children find symbolic solutions to old conflicts.

- *Mastery.* Serial drawings tap into the healing potential of the psyche and help children master experiences of loss and trauma (Allan, 1978). The process or act of drawing gives children a container for unconscious impulses, enabling them to gain a sense of personal control. This brings about a sense of well-being and improved functioning.

- *Relationship enhancement.* Jung believed that the key ingredient in therapeutic change stems from the attachment between child and therapist. The process of drawing session after session, with an understanding, nonintrusive therapist bolsters the child's ego and heals psychological trauma. Allan (1978) wrote that the therapeutic relationship "activates or reactivates the inner feeling of being loved and cared for. Over the sessions, this external relationship slowly becomes internalized and the feelings of being loved begin to act within the child outside of the counseling sessions" (p. 227).

Description

Ages

Five years and up.

Materials

Paper (8½ × 11 inches), a pencil, or crayons.

Setting

The technique involves regular individual sessions with the child for a minimum of 15–20 minutes. If possible, sessions should take place at the same time each week and in the same setting. It is important to find the creative media that the child prefers to work with. Furthermore, it is important that a trusting alliance be established between the child and therapist before using the serial drawing technique.

Techniques

Following a nondirective approach, the therapist asks the child to "Draw a picture. Any picture that you want to do." As the child draws, the therapist does not ask questions but does respond briefly if the child asks questions. When the drawing is complete, the therapist might help the child process it by asking a few questions, such as "I wonder if you could tell me what is happening in this picture?" and "Does this picture tell a story?" However, the therapist does not take notes to make certain that the child will experience him/her as present and involved in the process. Allan (1978) highlighted that the process of drawing alone does not bring about healing in the child. Rather, the therapeutic relationship activates the self-healing archetype.

Variations

In a directive approach, the therapist gives the child specific images to draw related to his/her trauma. In a semidirective approach, the therapist asks the child to redraw a specific symbol already made in order to examine its meaning and possible healing power.

Empirical Findings

Shedler (2010) found support for psychodynamic and analytic therapies, concluding that these approaches may not only decrease symptoms and distress, but also develop inner resources and coping skills that lead to a more fulfilling life. He highlighted that these approaches foster meaningful relationships, heal emotional scars from childhood, and promote resilience and self-worth.

Applications

The serial drawing technique is a nonthreatening method that provides information about unconscious processes and a way for children to overcome them. It is a helpful approach for engaging children in treatment, helping nonverbal children communicate, and helping children work through, master, and heal from experiences associated with abuse, trauma, disasters, and other significant losses. In addition, the technique enables children with attachment issues to rework developmental challenges through the therapeutic relationship, a key element in the technique.

References

Allan, J. (1978). Serial drawing: A therapeutic approach with young children. *Canadian Counsellor, 12*(4), 223–228.

Allan, J. (1988). *Inscapes of the child's world: Jungian counseling in schools and clinics.* Dallas, TX: Spring.

Allan, J., & Levin, S. (1993). Born on my bum: Jungian play therapy. In T. Kottman & C. Schaefer (Eds.), *Play therapy: A casebook for practitioners* (pp. 209–243). Northvale, NJ: Jason Aronson.

Allan, J. B. (1977). *Serial drawing: A therapeutic approach with young children.* Paper presented at the annual meeting of World Federation for Mental Health Congress, Vancouver, BC.

Shedler, J. (2010). The efficacy of psychodynamic psychotherapy. *American Psychologist, 65*(2) 98–109.

30

Collage

Collage is the twentieth century's greatest innovation.
—ROBERT MOTHERWELL

Introduction

Collage is an arrangement of materials or objects that are glued onto a surface to make a theme. Collage has been used since paper was invented in China around 200 B.C.E. but was not considered an art form until the cubist movement in the beginning of the 20th century. Pablo Picasso and Georges Braque coined the term *collage* from the French verb *coller*, which means "to glue." They used the term to describe art pieces made from pasting newsprint, fabric, rope, colored paper, and similar objects onto a larger surface. Artists throughout Europe used collage during this time.

One of the founders of the dada movement, Jean (Hans) Arp created "chance collages" by standing above a large sheet of paper, dropping bits of colored paper on it, and gluing the squares wherever they fell. This process freed Arp's artistic expression. Another dadaist, Kurt Schwitters incorporated paper, newspaper, advertisements, and waste materials to make three-dimensional collages that he called assemblages. Schwitters demonstrated that beauty could be made out of anything. Max Ernst, an artist associated with the dada and surrealist movements, was one of the first artists to apply Freud's theories to his creative expression. Ernst used his dream imagery in an attempt to create from the subconscious. His early experiences and primal emotions were the subject of his "collage novels" made from journals, novel illustrations, and catalogues. Years later, in the 1970s, collage was introduced as a technique for helping individuals in therapy.

Rationale

Collage making is a fun, engaging activity enjoyed by children of all ages. It does not require artistic ability. This makes collage less threatening and more accessible for children who lack artistic talent or confidence. The therapeutic benefits of collage making include:

- *Self-expression.* Collage making is a projective technique that fosters communication of subconscious thoughts and feelings. While choosing materials to include on a collage, children have the opportunity to explore memories, needs, wishes, and hopes. This process increases verbal communication and imparts understanding and insight.

- *Enjoyment.* Children enjoy cutting, pasting, and creating. Doing so increases a state of calm and openness. Creativity is also associated with a sense of well-being and self-esteem.

- *Externalization.* Collage making provides children with visual images of internal experiences, feelings, and relationships. This gives them the distance needed to look at their difficulties, achieve clarity, and explore ways to handle difficulties.

- *Competence.* The process of cutting and pasting images and materials to make a collage produces a sense of pride and competence. Children gain esteem from the finished product, which can be examined from session to session to track themes, changes, and progress.

Description

Ages

Four years and up.

Techniques

Collage making is a simple technique that involves four basic steps.

1. Decide what surface the child will use to make the collage. Large sheets of card stock, cardboard, paper bags, and shoe boxes are often used.

2. Gather scissors, tape, glue and/or glue sticks, crayons, markers, paints, and a variety of materials to foster self-expression. These can include construction paper, tissue paper, newspaper, magazine pictures, words, wallpaper, stickers, photographs, postcards, yarn, ribbon, cloth with various textures, lace, drawings, and products from nature such as leaves, flower petals, and seashells.

3. Provide directions. The therapist may suggest a specific theme or simply allow children to create a collage of their choosing. Themes for collage making often include values, poetry, dreams, goals, strengths, and memories.

4. Help children process the collage. Ask children to talk about the items they chose for their collage, what they see in it, and related feelings.

Variations

Memory Box

The use of collage to decorate memory boxes provides a means for children to free associate and process feelings about losses. The opportunity to make a memory box with images from magazines, photos, words, drawings, cards, and craft supplies gives children ages 5 years and up concrete reminders of their loved one and a way to hold on to positive memories.

Bag of Tricks

Cangelosi (1997) introduced the bag of tricks to help children ages 5 years and up during the termination phase of treatment. This technique involves giving children a brown paper bag to decorate/collage with pictures from magazines, drawings, and craft supplies. Children then fill the bag with magazine clippings, drawings, and words that portray tricks or coping skills that they learned in therapy. The bag reminds children of their outer originality and internal resources and promotes a sense of competence.

Scrapbook

Scrapbooking is an enjoyable, nonthreatening activity appropriate for children ages 5 years and up. Using collage to make personal books frees children to explore aspects of their relationships and internal worlds. Scrapbooks can be used for specific populations (Williams & Lent, 2008) or as a generic tool for self-exploration.

Nightmare Box

Hickey (2001) developed the nightmare box to help children ages 6–12 years overcome nightmares, fears, and worries about sleep. The technique involves having children collage a representation of their nightmare on the inside and outside of a box. The child then plays with and/or alters the box to make it less frightening.

Family Collage

In this technique, children ages 4 years and up are provided with various colors of construction paper and a glue stick. They are asked to choose a color to reflect the background (climate) of their family. They then tear shapes of colored paper to represent themselves and each family member. The shapes are glued onto the background as the child chooses. The therapist does not interpret the creation to the child. However, information about the background, presence or absence of family members and their placement, provides valuable clinical information (Shepard, 2003).

Empirical Findings

Meguro, Ishizaki, and Meguro (2009) found collage to be a promising technique for accessing the personal world of patients with dementia. Analysis of patients' collages showed spiritual images in the early stage and family images in the later stage of dementia.

Applications

Collage is a nonthreatening technique that is helpful for people of various ages and diagnostic categories. Its projective quality makes collage a particularly useful technique for children who have difficulty with verbal expression. Collage is helpful for addressing issues related to depression, anxiety, and adjustment issues involving losses, separation, and transitions. It can also be used to help children contain feelings rather than act them out. The collage technique can be applied in work with individuals, groups, and families.

References

Cangelosi, D. (1997). *Saying goodbye in child psychotherapy: Planned, unplanned and premature endings.* Northvale, NJ: Jason Aronson.

Hickey, D. A. (2001). The nightmare box: Empowering children through dreamwork. In H. G. Kaduson & C. E. Schaefer (Eds.), *101 more favorite play therapy techniques* (pp. 141–145). Northvale, NJ: Jason Aronson.

Meguro, M., Ishizaki, J., & Meguro, K. (2009). Collage technique may provide new perspectives for Alzheimer patients by exploring messages from their inner world. *Dementia Neuropsychology, 3*(4), 299–302.

Shepard, J. S. (2003). The family collage. In H. G. Kaduson & C. E. Schaefer (Eds.), *101 favorite play therapy techniques* (Vol. 3, pp. 3–6). Lanham, MD: Jason Aronson.

Williams, K., & Lent, J. (2008). Scrapbooking as an intervention for grief recovery. *Journal of Creativity in Mental Health, 3*(4), 455–467.

31

Painting

Painting is self-discovery. Every good artist paints what he is.
—JACKSON POLLOCK

Introduction

Cave dwellers as far back as 30,000–10,000 B.C.E. made the first paintings. Pre-historic artists initially painted with their fingers but later used pigment crayons and brushes made of animal hair. They also used reeds or hollowed bones to blow paint onto walls. Several different combinations of materials were used to make colored paints—for example, clay ochre was used to make red, yellow, and brown, and manganese or charcoals were used to make black. Pigments were grinded into a fine powder and mixed with cave water, animal fats, vegetable juice, blood, or urine to help it stick to the rock surface. Stone Age paintings commonly depicted hunting scenes; arrangements of animals such as bison, horses, reindeer, and mammoths; or abstract symbols such as dots, lines, and zigzags. Humans were rarely painted. The purpose of cave paintings is still unknown but some historians believe that they were purely decorative. Others argue that they were a form of communication. Still others believe cave paintings were made by shamans for ceremonial reasons—such as social, supernatural, or religious rituals (Encyclopedia of Stone Age Art, n.d.).

Painting was also common among ancient Egyptians. They painted on the walls of burial chambers using watercolor paints or cut outlines into walls, and painted the designs with watercolor washes. Paintings often recorded events in the deceased person's life.

With the rise of Christianity in the first century C.E., art became an important medium for teaching the principles of the church. Leaders of the church commissioned artists to decorate the walls of churches with frescoes, mosaics, and panel paintings to convey the teachings of Christianity. This made painting a popular medium, a respected career, and a form of communication.

Children have also enjoyed painting since pr-historic times. Researchers have revealed that children as young as 2 years decorated cave walls with finger flutings at least 13,000 years ago, creating simple lines as well as symbolic shapes. One cavern had so many children's flutings that researchers described it as a "playpen," for prehistoric children's recreation or rituals. However, it was not until 1938 that Dr. R. F. Shaw observed the effectiveness of finger painting for helping children overcome inhibitions and express fantasies. Since that time, painting has been considered one of the most useful techniques for working with children in clinical settings.

Rationale

Painting is an engaging activity with myriad therapeutic benefits:

• *Self-expression.* Painting is a projective technique that allows children to express their conscious feelings and emotional experiences more deeply than with words. It can provide access to unconscious fantasies and self-discovery.

• *Overcoming resistance.* Painting is an excellent tool for relaxing defenses and helping children overcome inhibitions and engage in treatment. In addition, providing children with the opportunity to use paints conveys a message of trust and shows the child that the therapist is interested in getting to know him/her. This serves as a building block for establishing a trusting relationship.

• *Creative thinking.* Painting helps children look at situations in a new, creative way. It forces them to make decisions regarding colors used, strokes applied, placement, and content. This helps them explore personal preferences and develop an individualized style for expressing themselves.

• *Fantasy.* Painting allows children to create and play with images. It frees them to make characters, places, and events, which gives them a way to compensate for difficulties in their real life. This promotes a sense of mastery and empowerment.

• *Self-esteem.* Learning to paint gives children a sense of pride and accomplishment. In addition, the response they get from others regarding their work bolsters their confidence and self-esteem. Because there is no right way in the arts, children who paint gain satisfaction from their unique artistic style. This is especially helpful for children who are perfectionists and those who lack confidence in their artistic abilities.

• *Stress relief.* The act of painting provides a comforting place for children and a respite from stress. It gives them time away from problems and restores resources for coping. Describing spin art, Hutchinson (2012) wrote: "In the creating of the art I noticed that clients relaxed, calmed, and had a centered focus. Watching the paint spin around and change has a somewhat hypnotic aspect to it."

Description

Ages

Painting can be used with children ages 2 years and up. The only requirement is that the child not put paint in his/her mouth. In general, younger children work best with large paper and broad paintbrushes. It is also helpful to use an easel with young children. Children ages 6–12 years show decreasing interest in tempera paints as they get older and an increasing interest in felt pens, colored pencils, and watercolors.

Materials

Paints, papers, brushes, smock.

Techniques

Finger Painting

Arlow and Kadis (1993) attempted to integrate finger painting in therapy, using it as a source of fantasies and free associations. Finger paints and paper are made available and the child is given free rein to paint whatever he/she wishes. Alternately, the therapist directs the child to paint a picture of "something important to you, or of a dream." When the painting is complete, the child is first asked to tell a story of the painting and then to discuss if there is anything about the painting that reminds him/her of real life. Arlow and Kadis highlighted the importance of observing how the child engages in finger painting by focusing on "the rate and rhythm of his work, the colors he employs, types of lines, and so forth" (p. 206).

Spin Art

Hutchinson (2012) introduced spin art as a therapeutic tool for children of any age. Using a battery-operated spin-art machine, card stock, and washable paints, the child places the colors he/she wishes onto the paper and watches them spin into a unique piece of art. Hutchinson noted that spin art can be used as a directive activity in which the therapist assigns a different feeling to each of the paint colors and encourages the child to discuss a time he/she felt that emotion while using it. In addition, the child can be asked to share one thing that happened since the previous session for each color of paint used. The technique can be adapted for family sessions by asking each member to take a turn adding a paint color to the work in progress and discussing how everyone adds something to the family.

Marble Painting

This technique, for children of any age, requires paper, paint, and several marbles. First, a piece of paper is placed on a rimmed cookie sheet or on the bottom of a shirt box. Several blobs of different-colored paint are dabbed onto the paper. Finally, the marbles are placed on the paper and the tray or box is tilted so that they roll around and create tracks in the paint.

Empirical Findings

Bar-Sela, Atid, Danos, Gabay, and Epelbaum (2007) examined the effects of watercolor painting on depression, anxiety, and fatigue levels in cancer patients undergoing chemotherapy. Sixty cancer patients participated in once-weekly art therapy sessions (painting with water-based paints). Nineteen patients participated in more than four sessions (intervention group) and 41 patients participated in fewer than two sessions (participant group). The Hospital Anxiety and Depression Scale (HADS) and the Brief Fatigue Inventory (BFI) were completed before every session, relating to the previous week. Results showed that BFI scores were lower in the intervention group than the participant group. In the intervention group, the median HADS score for depression was 9 at the beginning and 7 after the fourth appointment, showing a notable benefit of painting.

Applications

Painting is a versatile technique that can be used for children and adolescents of all ages with a wide variety of presenting problems. Since it is a projective tool, painting is especially helpful for shy, anxious, depressed, and inhibited children; individuals who have difficulty verbalizing feelings; and those who benefit from the escape that painting provides. Painting is a great way to start therapy because it relaxes defenses and provides a wealth of diagnostic information for therapists.

References

Arlow, J. A., & Kadis, A. (1993). Finger painting. In C. E. Schaefer & D. M. Cangelosi (Eds.), *Play therapy techniques* (pp. 161–175). Northvale, NJ: Jason Aronson.

Bar-Sela, G., Atid, L., Danos, S., Gabay, N., & Epelbaum, R. (2007). Art therapy improved depression and influenced fatigue levels in cancer patients on chemotherapy. *Psycho-Oncology, 16*(11), 980–984.

Encyclopedia of Stone Age Art. (n.d.). Stone Age cave painting prehistoric characteristics, origins, history, ideas. Retrieved from *www.visual-arts-cork.com/prehistoric/cave-painting. htm.*

Hutchinson, L. (2012). Using spin art in play therapy. Retrieved from *http://blog.playdrhutch. com/2012/10/4/using-spin-art.*

Shaw, R. F. (1938). *Finger painting.* Boston: Little, Brown.

32

Dance/Movement Play

Movement is the medium in which we live our lives.
—MARIAN CHACE

Maybe the Hokey Pokey really is what it is all about.
—ANONYMOUS

Introduction

Dance/movement therapy (DMT) is based on the idea that the body, mind, and spirit are interconnected. The American Dance Therapy Association (ADTA), founded in 1966, defined dance/movement therapy as "The psychotherapeutic use of movement as a process which furthers the emotional, cognitive, physical and social integration of the individual" (*www.adta.org*). Dance has been used as a healing ritual throughout history. It has served to enhance fertility, cure the ill, and mourn the dead. It has also been a source of entertainment in cultures throughout the world.

In the latter part of the 19th century, Europeans and Americans realized that dance had an effect on the dancer, bringing about changes in mood and affect. Marian Chace, often called the "Grand Dame" of DMT, was first to introduce the idea of DMT. Recognizing that her students were more interested in the emotions they expressed in dance than in the technique, she began to use dance for self-expression. This led to Chace becoming a member of the staff of St. Elizabeths Hospital in Washington, DC, where she offered "Dance for Communication," which was the start of a new mental health profession called DMT. When the ADTA was founded in 1966, Chace served as the first president. Since that time, the use of dance and other movement techniques have expanded for use with all age groups in hospitals, schools, and private practices.

Dance/movement play therapy (DMPT) is an integrated approach that blends the theories and techniques of play therapy with those of DMT. The intervention adds to DMT the distinctive qualities of play therapy—for example, spontaneity,

150

creativity, props, fantasy, games, silliness, mirth, and laughter—so as to enhance healing (Teichart, 2013). It involves expressing oneself playfully and metaphorically through the movement of one's body. DMPT is one model of integrated play therapy, a multitheoretical approach that is widely practiced throughout the world (Drewes, Bratton, & Schaefer, 2011).

Rationale

DMPT has many therapeutic benefits, including:

- *Diagnostic understanding.* Playful movement helps therapists obtain an understanding of children's inhibitions, how and where they hold stress, and the ways in which social/emotional issues affect them physiologically.
- *Self-expression.* It provides the opportunity to metaphorically express or dramatize thoughts and feelings that are difficult to communicate verbally.
- *Overcoming resistance.* Children are naturally more active than adults. They enjoy hopping, skipping, dancing, and other playful activities that serve to relax their defenses, help them relate to the therapist, and engage in treatment.
- *Catharsis.* Playful movement helps children release negative feelings associated with losses, injustices, separations, and transitions. This reduces anxiety and depression and frees children to live lives that are more carefree. It also helps them tolerate frustration better because they are no longer pent up with upsetting emotions.
- *Positive emotion.* Playful activities trigger laughter, joy, and mirth, which release endorphins that are known as the brain's feel-good neurotransmitters. Positive affect increases energy and optimism, reduces tension, and helps people stay calm in stressful situations.
- *Self-esteem.* Fun movement can increase self-confidence and lower the symptoms associated with depression and anxiety. It can also improve sleep, decreases stress, and gives children a sense of command over their body and life.
- *Game play.* Many games such as Twister and Red Light, Green Light involve the use of movement. These games increase social skills such as taking turns, playing fairly, and gracious winning and losing. They teach children that working cooperatively makes playing fun and fosters enjoyable friendships.

Description

Dance and movement can be incorporated into play therapy in a nonstructured, spontaneous way or by introducing specific play techniques to address children's clinical needs.

Ages

Two years and up.

Techniques

Dance Painting

Lite and Segal (2010) introduced this technique to reduce anxiety in children ages 2 years and up. Materials needed include mural or craft paper, washable paint, pans (for the paint), and tape. The therapist paints the bottom of the child's feet with the color he/she chooses, turns on music, and lets the child dance freely and playfully on the paper. The therapist can choose to play relaxing or energizing music depending on the child's needs.

Stomping Feet and Bubble Popping

Wunderlich (1997) introduced this technique for young children as a tool for expressing anger and frustration. The child's feet are outlined and colored. The therapist then discusses the importance of letting anger out and how this can be done by stomping in place on the drawing of the child's feet. The therapist also explains that the child will know anger is out when he/she feels better and the bottoms of his/her feet feel warm. After the child stomps, the therapist helps the child process how he/she feels differently and the child draws a mad face at the top of the shoe and a happy face at the bottom. Wunderlich also used bubble wrap to help children get rid of angry feelings. He found that most children are less angry after popping 10 bubbles with their fingers. We have also found it helpful to tape bubble wrap on the floor and let children gleefully stomp away their anger until all the bubbles have popped.

Scarf Story (Kaduson & Schaefer, 1997)

In this technique children take turns playfully and spontaneously moving under a large scarf held by the group. The therapist tells a story about a character that engages in various physical movements. At different points in the story the scarf is raised and the child under the scarf mimics and acts out the silly movements of the story character as they are being narrated by the therapist. Later the child describes what the story character may be feeling and thinking during the moves.

Hula Hoops

A thousand years ago children in Greece would roll bamboo circles on the ground with sticks, and spin the hoops around their waist. Therapists are using hula hoops today with individual and groups of children as a playful form of dance and movement. The activity tends to lift children's spirits, tone their body, and build mental focus.

Follow the Leader

Harvey (1990) developed the dynamic play therapy model, which integrated dance, movement, play, and other expressive arts. One technique is follow the leader in which parents and child take turns following the moves led by each other, including such movements as jumping, crawling, and rolling on the floor, and climbing over a stack of pillows. These and other playful, physical interactions can be used to foster a child's attachment to his/her parents.

Freeze Dancing

In this activity, children in group therapy dance to music. When the therapist stops the music everyone freezes in place. Children dance slowly to slow songs and quickly to fast songs.

Wacky Dancing

In group therapy, the therapist puts on some fun music and then starts to dance. The group members have to follow his/her dance moves exactly, no matter how wacky. After about 30 seconds the therapist calls out a child's name and that child begins to make up his/her own dance routine that the rest of the group must follow.

Feeling Movement

Ask the child to make a movement (or gesture) to represent a feeling, such as anger or fear.

Empirical Findings

This technique is in need of empirical research.

Applications

Moving and dancing in a playful way is a beneficial, enjoyable, and developmentally appropriate activity for children. It is nonthreatening, loosens defenses, and engages children in treatment because it is a fun activity. It helps reduce depression by activating endorphin levels, it reduces anxiety by providing a release, and it aids shy and inhibited children to express themselves. Children with hyperactivity and behavior difficulties often find it difficult to sit still and talk directly to a therapist. However, they enjoy physical activities, which can expend energy and reduce their level of physical arousal.

References

Drewes, A., Bratton, S., & Schaefer, C. E. (Eds.). (2011). *Integrative play therapy*. Hoboken, NJ: Wiley.

Harvey, S. (1990). Dynamic play therapy: An integrated expressive art approach to the family therapy of young children. *Arts in Psychotherapy, 17*, 239–246.

Kaduson, H. G., & Schaefer, C. E. (Eds.). (1997). *101 favorite play therapy techniques*. Northvale, NJ: Jason Aronson.

Lite, L., & Segal, S. (2010, September 10). Dance painting reduces stress and eases anxiety in preschoolers. Retrieved from *www.stressfreekids.com/3923/painting-reduces-stress*.

Teichart, A. (2013). *The phenomenon of play within a dance/movement setting with adults*. Unpublished master's thesis, Columbia College, Chicago.

Wunderlich, C. (1997). Stomping feet and bubble popping. In H. G. Kaduson & C. E. Schaefer (Eds.), *101 favorite play therapy techniques* (pp. 283–285). Northvale, NJ: Jason Aronson.

33

Draw a Family

When the child can take the "picture" in his head and transfer it
onto a piece of paper, it becomes an object for action.
—NANCY BOYD WEBB

Introduction

Goodenough (1926) introduced the idea of using human figure drawings to assess developmental maturity. Since that time, a variety of drawing techniques have been developed for assessment and therapeutic purposes. Often, children are able to convey in their drawings thoughts and feelings that they cannot express in speech or writing. Hulse (1951, 1952) was the first to use children's drawings as a means of providing insight into a child's perception of his/her family relationships. The understanding of family dynamics is critical for formulating an effective treatment plan for most children.

Rationale

The draw-a-family technique has projective and healing qualities that benefit children in a variety of ways:

• *Working alliance.* Drawing activities are helpful for resistant children and those who have a hard time talking about feelings. In addition, the projective qualities of the draw-a-family technique provide therapists with a snapshot of children's relationships, which fosters an understanding of the child's perceptions and needs. This clinical insight enables the therapist to be attuned and responsive to the child and fosters a trusting relationship.

• *Positive emotion.* Children of all ages find drawing enjoyable and relaxing.

155

In addition, drawing can result in short-term improved mood (Drake & Winner, 2013).

• *Communication.* The draw-a-family technique provides children with a nonverbal way to convey feelings, perceptions, attitudes, and needs about family members. These are revealed in indicators such as size, style, facial and bodily features, and placement.

Description

Ages

Six to 12 years.

Materials

Pencil and a piece of blank white paper.

Techniques

The simple instruction to the child is "Draw a picture of your family for me, including yourself." The therapist then asks the child to identify the figures and discuss whatever he/she would like to say about the drawing. Qualitative aspects such as the relative size of the figures, the distance between figures, and their distribution on the paper are noted. In addition, the order in which family members were drawn, the force of the child's pencil stroke, shading and coloring, and omissions or exaggerations of family members (including the child) are noteworthy (Klepsch & Logie, 1982).

Variations

Child and Parent Family Drawings

Shearn and Russel (1970) expanded the draw-a-family technique by obtaining family drawings from children as well as one or more parents. They found that comparing drawings provides a more specific understanding of the feelings, perceptions, roles, and dynamics of family members as well as the overall family climate.

Family Drawing/Storytelling

In this technique (Roosa, 1981, p. 270) the child is first asked to draw a picture of his/her family. Then the therapist asks the child to "Make up a story about what your family is doing in the picture. Also, tell what happened before this, how each person feels, and how the story ends."

Family Drawing Interview

For children who are particularly reticent or verbally limited, Grunes (1979, p. 15) recommended asking the child a list of questions about his/her family drawing, such as "Who is the strongest? Which person likes Daddy the most?" If needed, the child can respond by pointing to the figure in his/her drawing.

Kinetic Family Drawing

Burns and Kaufman (1970) introduced a variation of the draw-a-family technique, called the kinetic family drawing (KFD). It has become a widely used diagnostic tool for children ages 6–16 years. Unlike the draw-a-family technique that focuses on stationary figures, the instructions and analysis of KFDs address action and the way a family functions. Instructions to the child are "Draw a picture of everyone in your family, including yourself, doing something. Try to draw whole people, not cartoon or stick people. Remember, make everyone doing something—some kind of action" (Burns & Kaufman, 2013, p. 5). When the drawing is complete, the child is asked to identify each person and what he/she is doing. This provides more information about the child's perceptions of family dynamics, physical inter-actions, and emotional relationships.

The KFD has a comprehensive scoring system that addresses four major cat-egories: action; physical characteristics; distance, barrier, and positions; and styles. Actions refer to the content or theme of the drawing (e.g., cooperation, nurtur-ance, tension). Physical characteristics refer to facial expressions, inclusion of body parts, size of figures, and so on. Distance, barrier, and positions involve the direc-tion that figures face and the distance between them. Finally, styles refer to the way in which the child organizes figures on the paper.

Sensory/Kinetic Hand Family Drawing (Filley, 2003)

This technique requires paper and markers, crayons, or other writing materials. First, the therapist or parent/caregiver traces the child's hand onto a piece of paper. On each finger of his/her hand tracing, the child identifies one family member by drawing a picture of the person, representing the person with a symbol, or writ-ing his/her name. At the wrist, the child can write or draw other important people in his/her life or something that connects the family together (e.g., sports, music, arguing). In the palm or "heart" of the hand, the child draws a symbol, something the family does together, and so on. When used with families or parent–child dyads, each family member completes his/her own hand tracing. This technique can be adapted by using paint, pudding, or clay to enhance sensory experiences.

Make a Family Drawing

Kaduson (2003) created this technique for children with fine motor difficul-ties, perfectionism, and children reluctant to draw because they feel they are not good artists. It is ideal for very young children who lack drawing skills. Before the intake, the therapist cuts out pictures of items that children draw in family drawings. These would include faces, shirts, pants, skirts, dresses, shoes, sneakers, tables, chairs, balls, and so on. The focus is on choosing a variety of expressions and styles to provide children with options and a means for what they want to convey. The pictures are presented to the child in boxes so that most of the pictures can be seen when the child looks at the box. A piece of paper (11 × 14 inches) and a glue stick are then provided and the child is instructed to create a picture of his/her family. This technique can be used with groups and families provided that enough cut-out items are available.

Family Interaction Diagram

Truax (2003) introduced this technique for children ages 6–12 years. The child is given drawing paper and colored markers, pencils, or crayons and is instructed to draw each of his/her family members with names underneath. Children living in more than one family are instructed to fold the paper in half and draw each family group in a separate column. The child then chooses a color that stands for people getting along really well and draws a line between all the people who get along well. Separate colors are used to represent not getting along well, fight a lot, and so on. This technique is especially useful for foster children, children of divorce, and those with large and/or complex family situations.

Draw-a-Group Test

Assessment tools similar to the draw-a-family technique have been used to evaluate and understand children's key relationships with individuals outside of the family. Hare and Hare (1956) introduced the draw-a-group test to assess the roles and dynamics of children's friendships. In this technique, the child draws a picture of the peers he/she enjoys playing with and the activity that he/she likes to do with them. A similar tool, the draw-a-classroom technique, was introduced by Kutnick (1978) to evaluate and understand children's perceptions and experiences about school. In this technique, the child draws a picture of a classroom with people in it. Discussion and analysis of the drawing focuses on people and their actions, the classroom and objects in it, and the depiction of the teacher (Klepsch & Logie, 1982).

Empirical Findings

   1. Daren (1975) compared family drawings of 239 African American, Puerto Rican, and Caucasian family members referred to a psychiatric clinic. The examiner scored the drawings for size, detail, and number of family members. Results showed significant size differences among the groups. In particular, the African American participants' drawings showed larger mother figures than the other groups. In all groups, children often drew larger families than they had.

2. Piperno, Di Biasi, and Levi (2007) discovered that physically and/or sexually abused children, ages 5–10 years, were likely to exclude their primary caregiver from their family drawings.

3. Gardano (1988) contrasted the family drawings of children with alcoholic fathers with the drawings of a matched control group. Children with alcoholic fathers drew family members of similar sizes with significantly more distance between them as compared with the control group, who drew family members that varied in size and were closer together. There was a highly significant difference in the distance between the mother and father in the experimental group, whose drawings demonstrated a general sense of disengagement. In addition, the control group drew significantly larger mothers.

4. Gross and Hayne (1998) examined the effect that drawing has on young children's verbal responses about their emotional experiences. Children were asked to draw and then tell or to just tell about a time when they felt happy, sad, scared, or angry. Children given the opportunity to draw and tell reported significantly more information about emotional experiences than children who did not have the opportunity to draw before telling. These findings suggest that drawing tends to increase young children's ability to talk about emotion-laden experiences.

Applications

The draw-a-family technique is appropriate for children with all types of presenting problems. Because it is a projective tool, this technique enables children to convey feelings, emotions, and perceptions that they may not be aware of or that they cannot express verbally. It is very helpful for children who are nonverbal, shy, or inhibited, and those who conceal feelings.

The draw-a-family technique is also a helpful diagnostic tool, especially useful during the intake or beginning phase of treatment. Observing children's approach to the task and noting the content of family drawings provides therapists with an understanding of children's needs and struggles. This information is useful for developing a trusting relationship and for treatment planning. For instance, if a child conveys that parents are overbearing in his/her drawing (and if this information is backed up in the history and/or clinical observations), a client-centered approach for treatment may be beneficial. Conversely, if the child conveys a need for structure and guidance, a more directive, structured treatment approach may be indicated.

References

Burns, R. C., & Kaufman, S. H. (1970). *Kinetic family drawings (K-F-D)*. New York: Brunner/Mazel.

Burns, R. C., & Kaufman, S. H. (2013). *Actions, styles, and symbols in kinetic family drawings (K-F-D): An interpretive manual*. New York: Brunner/Mazel.

Daren, S. (1975). An empirical evaluation of the validity of the draw-a-family test. *Journal of Clinical Psychology, 31,* 542–546.

Drake, J. E., & Winner, E. (2013). How children use drawing to regulate their emotions. *Cognition and Emotion, 27*(3), 512–520.

Filley, D. K. (2003). Sensory/kinetic hand family drawing. In H. G. Kaduson & C. E. Schaefer, *101 favorite play therapy techniques* (Vol. 3, pp. 42–45). Northvale, NJ: Jason Aronson.

Gardano, A. (1988). *A revised scoring method for kinetic family drawings and its implication to the evaluation of family structure with an emphasis on children from alcoholic families.* Unpublished doctoral dissertation, George Washington University.

Goodenough, F. L. (1926). *Measurement of intelligence by drawings.* New York: Harcourt, Brace & World.

Gross, J., & Hayne, H. (1998). Drawing facilitates children's verbal reports of emotionally laden events. *Journal of Experimental Psychology: Applied, 4,* 163–179.

Grunes, W. (1979). The Grunes' "which one" interview procedure. *Journal of Learning Disabilities, 12,* 146–149.

Hare, A. P., & Hare, R. T. (1956). The draw-a-group test. *Journal of Genetic Psychology, 89,* 51–59.

Hulse, W. (1952). Childhood conflict expressed through family drawings. *Journal of Projective Techniques, 16*(1), 66–79.

Hulse, W. C. (1951). The emotionally disturbed child draws his family. *Quarterly Journal of Child Behavior, 3,* 152–174.

Kaduson, H. G. (2003). Make a family drawing. In H. G. Kaduson & C. E. Schaefer (Eds.), *101 favorite play therapy techniques* (Vol. 3, pp. 93–95). Northvale, NJ: Jason Aronson.

Klepsch, M., & Logie, L. (1982). *Children draw and tell: An introduction to the projective uses of children's human figure drawings.* New York: Brunner/Mazel.

Kutnick, P. (1978). Children's drawings of their classrooms: Development and social maturity. *Child Study Journal, 8,* 175–185.

Piperno, F., Di Biasi, G., & Levi, G. (2007). Evaluation of family drawings of physically and sexually abused children. *European Child and Adolescent Psychiatry, 16,* 389–397.

Roosa, L. (1981). The family drawing/storytelling technique: An approach to assessment of family dynamics. *Elementary School Guidance and Counseling, 15,* 269–272.

Shearn, C. R., & Russel, K. R. (1970). Use of the family drawing technique for studying parent–child interaction. *Journal of Projective Techniques and Personality Assessment, 33*(1), 35–44.

Truax, K. (2003). Family interaction diagram. In H. G. Kaduson & C. E. Schaefer (Eds.), *101 favorite play therapy techniques* (Vol. 3, pp. 93–95). Northvale, NJ: Jason Aronson.

34

Family Sculpting

Every word, facial expression, gesture, or action on the part of a
parent gives the child some message about self-worth. It is sad that so
many parents don't realize what messages they are sending.
                                                      —Virginia Satir

Introduction

Family sculpting is a family therapy technique that is widely used to assess family
dynamics. Its roots go back to Minuchin's (1974) thinking about the importance
of observing and manipulating the spatial closeness and distance among family
members. It can provide insight into family structure issues, including boundaries, cohesion, alliances, hierarchy, and alienation. As a tool in play therapy, family
sculpting helps children transform feelings and perceptions, which are difficult to
express, into an external diagram or sculpture (Simon, 1972).

Rationale

Family sculpting is a powerful assessment tool and a valuable aid to therapy. It
provides a number of therapeutic benefits, including:

• *Self-expression*. This technique enables children to show their internal perceptions and experiences of their family in a tangible way. It provides a visual
representation of emotional alliances and conflicts, and patterns of closeness, distance, restriction, nurturance, clinginess, inclusions, and exclusions within the
family system. This gives the therapist valuable information for treatment planning that most children cannot convey verbally or which would take an inordinate
amount of time to uncover.

• *Relationship enhancement*. The process of family sculpting can strengthen empathic connections within the family. Family members who see the sculpture gain an appreciation of how the child views the family, in a way that is much more powerful than words. This can foster understanding and promote communication and closer family relationships. When sculptures are done in group therapy, members of the group gain a new understanding of one another's feelings, situations, and struggles. They often provide support and alternate solutions to one another and may form closer relationships as a result of this process.

• *Conflict resolution.* The illustrative quality of family sculpting highlights problematic behaviors and can be a helpful tool for conflict resolution in families and among peers.

• *Power.* Family sculpting is empowering because it puts the child in charge of sculpting his/her own family experience. This is ego boosting for the child.

Description

Ages

Family sculpting in one form or another is appropriate for children ages 6 years and up. The only requirement is that children understand the directions.

Techniques

The child is told to create a family sculpture by physically placing family members together into a sculpture that reflects the present family situation or the typical way in which family members interact with one another. This is done by the child directing family members to assume specific postures, expressions, and distances between each other to convey the child's internal experience of family dynamics. Sometimes the initial sculpture could become a moving sculpture to show a sequence of interactions or events. Props may be used, such as a rope for the family to engage in a tug-of-war to illustrate members going in opposite directions.

Perkins (1999) described three general types of family sculpting. In the first, actual family members are used to form the sculpture during a family session. In the second, surrogates are used to represent family members as a part of group counseling where members take turns sculpting their families. Finally, in the third, symbolic representations of family members are used. These can include puppets, drawings of family members, miniature dolls, toys, or other creative art materials such as clay. Several symbolic family sculptures are described below.

Variations

Family Sculpting with Puppets

Haslam (2010) introduced this activity to help family members express feelings using a multisensory medium. Each family member gets a turn to choose a puppet that represents each person in the family and arrange the puppets to convey what things feel like in the family. The puppets can be close together, far apart, in the open, or hidden. After each person has sculpted the puppets, the therapist asks them to tell about the scene they created and describe feelings that exist among the puppets. In addition, the other family members are asked to reflect about the sculpture and the feelings and thoughts it prompted. Focus is exploratory and aimed at providing the family with a positive experience.

Clay Family Sculpting

In this technique, the child client designs a clay representation of each family member in a way that reflects that person's personality and role in the family. When all the sculptures are complete, the child places them in relation to each other, to convey relationships and interactions.

Kyebaek Family Sculpting

This technique involves the use of a specifically designed set of 17 hardwood figures resembling human figures and one pet. In this technique (Berry, Hurley, & Worthington, 1990), the child uses a grid board similar to a checkerboard and the small wooden figures to depict the distance among family members. Distance can be measured objectively as well as subjectively.

Family System Test (Gehring & Wyler, 1986)

The Family System Test uses a set of wooden dolls and a grid board for a child to portray typical or ideal family relations in terms of two dimensions: cohesion (emotional closeness) and hierarchy (power). It is a rapid, easy to administer, and engaging instrument that can be administered to individual children/adolescents, families, and extended families.

Bottom of Form

Empirical Findings

1. Berry and colleagues (1990) studied 31 families with at least one adolescent and two parents. They used the Kyebaek family sculpture technique (KFST) to assess emotional distance among family members and compared it with cohesion measured by the Family Adaptability and Cohesion Evaluation Scale III (FACES III). Results showed that KFST distance was significantly related to FACES III cohesion, supporting convergent validity for the KFST.

2. Gehring and Marti (1993) found that children in therapy, compared with children not in therapy, were less likely on the Family System Test to portray their families as being cohesive and moderately hierarchical or as having clear generational boundaries.

Applications

Family sculpting is a useful technique for assessing family dynamics in a wide range of child and adolescent clients. It allows the family structure to "quickly and dramatically become visible" (Hartman & Laird, 1983). The technique is beneficial for children with issues related to attachment, custody, and parental abuse or neglect. Family sculpting is especially helpful for children with poor verbal skills, limited insight, oppositional tendencies, and problematic family relationships.

References

Berry, J. T., Hurley, J. H., & Worthington, E. L. (1990). Empirical validity of the Kvebaek family sculpture technique. *American Journal of Family Therapy, 18*(1), 19–31.

Gehring, T., & Marti, D. (1993). The Family System Test: Differences in perception of family structure between nonclinical and clinical children. *Journal of Child Psychology, 34*(3), 363–372.

Gehring, T. M., & Wyler, I. L. (1986). Family System Test (FAST): A three-dimensional approach to investigate family relationships. *Child Psychiatry and Human Development, 16*, 235–248.

Hartman, A., & Laird, J. (1983). *Family-centered social work practice.* New York: Free Press.

Haslam, D. (2010). Family sculpting with puppets. In L. Lowenstein (Ed.), *Creative family therapy techniques: Play, art, and expressive therapies to engage children in family sessions* (pp. 138–141). Toronto: Champion Press.

Minuchin, S. (1974). *Family and family therapy.* London: Tavistock.

Perkins, M. R. (1999). An introduction to family sculpting, version 1.9. Retrieved from *https://sites.google.com/site/homepageformikeperkins/Home/family-sculpting.*

35

Musical Play

Where words fail, music speaks.
— HANS CHRISTIAN ANDERSEN

Introduction

From a very early age, children delight in making sounds with their voices and various objects. The therapeutic value of music has been recognized since ancient times. Ancient Egyptians used music for healing by chanting. Greek physicians used flutes and lyres to heal illness, and vibrations to improve digestion and induce sleep. Native Americans used a variety of drums, rattles, and vocal sounds in healing rituals. Thousands of years ago, Aristotle noted that music could stir strong emotions and purify the soul.

The earliest reference to music therapy appeared in 1789 in a magazine entitled *Music Physically Considered*. However, it was not until the end of World War I and World War II when musicians began to play for veterans suffering from physical and emotional trauma that the significance of music for emotional healing soared (American Music Therapy Association, 2015). Since that time, music has been used to soothe, stimulate, arouse, and engage individuals with a wide variety of clinical needs and presenting problems. It has been used in hospitals, schools, and private practices with children of all ages.

Bender and Woltman (1941) first introduced the idea of using music as an adjunct to play therapy, noting its value in nonverbal communication. In music play therapy, musical toys and instruments are provided for the child to enhance self-expression and communication. Unlike music therapy, which is a specialized field requiring significant training, music play therapy does not require that the therapist have such a musical background.

165

Rationale

Research shows that music provides access to emotions, fosters learning, and improves attention (Children's Music Workshop, 2014). In addition, children are naturally drawn to music and it has a number of therapeutic benefits when used in play therapy:

• *Overcoming resistance.* The use of familiar music and/or the presence of musical instruments in the playroom can help to relieve children's anxiety when starting treatment. This can serve to relax children's defenses and help the therapist to establish a working alliance.

• *Creative thinking.* Music enhances the ability to think creatively. It can challenge children to solve problems by imagining and playing with various solutions.

• *Self-expression.* Music provides a safe, enjoyable way for children to express feelings, thoughts, ideas, and preferences. It relieves inhibitions and builds confidence.

• *Positive emotion.* Singing, humming, or simply listening to music or exploring musical instruments fosters children's imaginations and eases the pressures of everyday life. In addition, use of soothing music serves as a tool for relaxation, stress management, and pain reduction.

• *Competence.* The inherent structure and emotional pull of music makes it a beneficial tool for teaching concepts and ideas (Merzenich, 2010). Research shows that connecting new information to familiar songs enhances children's ability to learn (Children's Music Workshop, 2014). Music is a fun mnemonic device that marks information and enhances memory and learning. Used in play therapy, music can help children remember discussions and learn new skills.

• *Executive functioning.* There is a causal link between music and spatial intelligence (the ability to perceive the world accurately and to form mental pictures). This ability allows children to visualize various elements that should go together and is critical for planning and problem solving (Children's Music Workshop, 2014).

• *Self-esteem.* Because music contributes to a feeling of self-efficacy related to learning new skills, it can have a positive effect on children's self-esteem. In addition, learning to play a musical instrument helps children conquer fears and contributes to a sense of mastery.

• *Relationship enhancement.* Use of music in group therapy can facilitate communication and enhance interpersonal relationships.

Description

Ages

Three years and up.

Materials

A variety of simple music-making objects, such as maracas, drums, bells, or shakers. Also helpful are a CD player or iPod port, toy microphones, and a selection of songs dealing with self-esteem, feelings, and friendships.

Techniques

Musical play techniques, which blend music and play, include various forms of music such as singing, humming, playing a musical instrument, composing a silly song, using background music, listening to lyrics, and or performing. Each of these techniques can be applied in the playroom for use with individuals, families, and groups. Carmichael (2002) suggested that play therapists display the musical materials and then structure the activity with a statement such as "Today, I thought you might like to play some music." The child is then free to play or sing whatever he/she wishes. Subsequently, a child may seek structure by wanting to play a certain instrument or sing a particular song (Moreno, 1985).

Variations

Song Games

Song games use song lyrics to guide the movements of a group of preschoolers in a fun way. Examples include "The Hokey Pokey"; "Head, Shoulders, Knees, and Toes"; and "I'm a Little Teapot." Song games promote executive functioning because the children have to move to a specific rhythm and synchronize the words to actions and the music.

Therapist-Created Song

Carmichael (2002) introduced the idea of making up a song for the child, singing it to him/her and inviting the child to change the lyrics or add more verses.

Music Painting

While listening to music, the child is asked to paint (or color) a picture of a thought or feeling that the music brings to mind.

Dancing Games

Play some music and have children dance very fast and very slowly. "Freeze danc-ing" can be fun as well and it can be made more challenging by asking the children to freeze in particular positions (e.g., hands up high).

Clapping Games

Rhythmic clapping strengths children's inhibitory control and cognitive flexibility. It has been popular with generations of children in many cultures.

Nondirective Music Play Therapy

Moreno (1985) developed this model for providing music play therapy, which inte-grates music therapy and the underlying philosophy and concepts of nondirective play therapy. The playroom is equipped with musical instruments and the child is given the opportunity to play out his/her feelings with them. Moreno believed that the duality of structure and nonstructure of musical instruments is beneficial in the therapeutic process. Instruments provide structure because of the limita-tions in tone and rhythm they produce—for example, piano keys must be pressed and flutes must be blown. Nonstructure is experienced by the variety of emotions expressed in the tones and rhythms. Moreno believed that change occurs when the child moves from exploring musical instruments to asking to learn melodies. He believed that the goal of treatment is reached when the child uses music outside of therapy for emotional expression.

Song Flute or Recorder

Freeman (1997) developed this technique as an adjuvant action that "aids, facili-tates, and enhances treatment" (p. 348). He highlighted that it helps to engage children in treatment, encourage interaction with the therapist, teach a new skill, foster self-esteem, and identify change and development. Materials needed include a song flute or recorder, Hoenack's *Let's Sing and Play Music Book* (1986), and an instruction book that the therapist reads before teaching the instrument to the child. The therapist starts by teaching the child how to hold the instrument, the B finger position, followed by the A finger position, and finally the G finger position. After minimal practice of the three notes (B, A, G) the child attempts to play the first song in Hoenack's music book and gradually progresses through the remain-ing songs in the book before learning the next note.

Empirical Findings

   1. Kim, Wigram, and Gold (2009) found that children with autism demon-strated more emotional expression and social engagement during music therapy sessions than in play sessions without music. In addition, these children responded to the therapist's requests more frequently during music therapy than in play sessions without music.

2. Hendon and Bohon (2008) reported that hospitalized children, ages 1–12 years, were happier during music therapy rather than play therapy.

3. In a study that involved 96 four-year-olds in joint music making, Kirschner and Tomasello (2010) showed that these children subsequently increased their spontaneous, cooperative, and helping behaviors.

4. In a recent review of research on musical play, Pound (2010) concluded that it promotes a wide range of adaptive behaviors, including social interactions, self-expression, emotion understanding, and self-regulation.

5. Loewy, Stewart, Dassler, Telsey, and Homel (2013) examined the effects of music on the vital signs, feeding, and sleep patterns of 272 premature babies. They studied the effects of three types of music: a lullaby selected and sung by the baby's parents; an "ocean disc" that mimics the sounds of the womb; and a Gato box, a drum-like instrument used to simulate two-tone heartbeat rhythms. The two instruments were played live by certified music therapists, who matched their music to the babies' breathing and heart rhythms. Findings showed that they all served to decrease heart rates. However, singing was the most effective. Singing also increased the amount of time babies remained quietly alert, lowered the parents' stress level, and enhanced bonding. The findings have implications for helping parents bond with an older child experiencing an attachment disorder.

Applications

Musical play is a helpful approach to treatment for children who enjoy music. It helps engage children and adolescents in treatment; enhances openness and communication in shy, anxious, nonverbal, and inhibited individuals; increases emotional expression and social responsiveness in children with Asperger's syndrome; decreases depression and anxiety; and aids in remembering life events. Musical play also promotes socialization, making it a useful resource for children with developmental delays and social skills deficits.

References

American Music Therapy Association. (2015). History of music therapy. Retrieved from *www. musictherapy.org/about/history*.

Bender, L., & Woltman, A. G. (1941). Play and psychotherapy. *Nervous Child*, *11*, 17–42.

Carmichael, K. (2002). Music play therapy. In C. E. Schaefer & D. M. Cangelosi (Eds.), *Play therapy techniques* (2nd ed.). Northvale, NJ: Jason Aronson.

Children's Music Workshop. (20014, November 29). Twelve benefits of music education. Retrieved from *www.childrensmusicworkshop.com/twelve-benefits-of-music-education*.

Freeman, R. W. (1997). The song flute or recorder. In H. G. Kaduson & C. E. Schaefer (Eds.), *101 favorite play therapy techniques* (pp. 347–352). Northvale, NJ: Jason Aronson.

Hendon, C., & Bohon, L. M. (2008). Hospitalized children's mood differences during play and music therapy. *Child: Care, Health, and Development, 34*(2), 141–144.

Hoenack, P. (1986). *Let's sing and play, book 1*. Bethesda, MD: Music for Young People.

Kim, J., Wigram, T., & Gold, C. (2009). Emotional, motivational, and interpersonal responsiveness of children with autism in improvisational music therapy. *Autism, 13*(4), 389–409.

Kirschner, S., & Tomasello, M. (2010). Joint music making promotes social behavior in 4-year-old children. *Evolution and Human Behavior, 31*(5), 354–364.

Loewy, J., Stewart, K., Dassler, A. M., Telsey, A., & Homel, P. (2013). The effects of music therapy on vital signs, feeding, and sleep in premature infants. *Pediatrics, 131*(5), 902–918.

Merzenich, K. (2010). Top 12 brain-based reasons why music as therapy works. *Neuroscience*. Retrieved from *http://blog.brainhq.com/2010/04/22/top-12-brain-based-reasons-why-music-as-therapy-works*.

Moreno, J. (1985). Music play therapy: An integrated approach. *Arts in Psychotherapy, 12*(1), 17–23.

Pound, L. (2010). Playing music. In J. Moyles (Ed.), *The excellence of play* (pp. 139–153). Maidenhead, UK: Open University Press.

Part Five

IMAGERY AND FANTASY TECHNIQUES

36

Guided Imagery

Introduction

The use of imagery in psychotherapy has a long history. Desoille (1945) was a pioneer who developed the method of "guided daydream" as a therapeutic tool in the 1920s. Desoille directed his patients, while in a state of relaxation, to close their eyes and actively daydream about themes such as approaching a threatening, archetypal figure. Images can be defined as mental representations of a sensory or perceptual-like experience that occurs in the absence of a stimulus that would produce the real experience (Richardson, 1969; Sherrod & Singer, 1984). Imagery is the art of making and manipulating images (e.g., forming mental pictures of a forest or seashore). The capacity to use imagery as a coping skill can be developed and encouraged by the therapist.

Rationale

- Imagery affords access to important events occurring early in life prior to the predominance of language.

- Images tend to bypass one's defenses, thus providing wider areas to explore in psychotherapy.

- In many cases, the therapeutic value of metaphors in guided imagery seems to produce therapeutic change in the absence of interpretations by the therapist or client insight (Desoille, 1961; Klinger, 1980).

IMAGERY RESCRIPTING AND REHEARSAL

Introduction

For many decades therapists have been helping children change the endings of their maladaptive stories, imagery, and dreams (Gardner, 1971). One recent variation of this approach for the treatment of childhood nightmares is the imagery rescripting and rehearsal technique.

Rationale

The rationale for this cognitive-behavioral technique is that images have stronger emotional and memory effects than verbal instruction. Also, creating and practicing a mastery ending to a scary dream eliminates the threatening content and changes the previous feelings of helplessness and vulnerability to feelings of power and control.

Description

Ages

Four to 8 years.

Techniques

This form of guided imagery involves helping a child rescript and thus create a more positive ending for a recurrent nightmare (Halliday, 1987; Krakow, 2001). During the day, the child is told that scary dreams are like movies that we make up for ourselves, that they are not real, and that we can change them to make them less scary. The child is then asked what he/she would like to happen in the dream so he/she wouldn't be scared. This process is like assertiveness training for the imagination.

Imagery rescripting is one part of the four-component nightmare relief therapy developed by Siegel (1998) and Krakow (2001). In this strategy, children are first given immediate emotional and physical *reassurance* by their parents so that they feel safe and comforted after the bad dream. The next day, *rescripting* is used by the parents to help the child to change some aspect of the bad dream to make it less scary and develop a sense of mastery over it—for example, one can make friends with the dream monster, or it can be tricked, chased away by a superhero, and generally made harmless. *Rehearsal* is the third step in which the child uses miniature, dream-related toys to act out and practice the new mastery ending. This playful practice lasts 10–20 minutes daily for 3 consecutive days or until a sense of control is achieved by the child. If the child is reluctant to practice at home, the therapist can play out a positive ending in the therapy sessions. In the final *resolution* phase of the approach, the parents and therapist seek to uncover and resolve any ongoing cause of the nightmare experience (e.g., bullying, abuse).

Variations

The book *How Zac Got His Z's: A Guide to Getting Rid of Nightmares* by child therapist Kerri Golding Oransky (2011), tells the story of a boy who learned a secret rescripting technique to successfully eliminate his nightmares. This book has received positive parent reviews.

Empirical Findings

I. To date, the imagery rescripting and rehearsal technique has received considerable research support for treating frequent nightmares in children, adolescents, and adults (Simard & Nielsen, 2009)—for example, St-Onge, Mercier, and De Koninck (2009) investigated the use of imagery rehearsal therapy (IRT) for 20 school-age children with moderate to severe nightmares. The children were randomly assigned to an IRT group or a wait-list control group. The IRT intervention significantly reduced the frequency of nightmares in the treated group compared with the wait-list group. This reduction was maintained over a 9-month follow-up period.

2. A meta-analysis conducted by Hansen, Hofling, Kroner-Barowik, Strangier, and Steil (2013) of the effectiveness of psychological treatments for chronic nightmares using imagery confrontation with nightmare content or imagery rescripting and rehearsal revealed high effect sizes for both interventions.

Applications

The imagery rescripting and rehearsal technique has been found particularly effective in reducing the frequency of nightmares in school-age children. It has also been found helpful in rescripting the trauma memories of children and adults suffering from PTSD (Casement & Swanson, 2012; Hackman, 2011).

Contraindications

Guided imagery should not be used in the absence of a trusting relationship with the therapist. More specifically, it can be harmful to clients who are freely dissociating or acutely psychotic.

GUIDED RELAXATION IMAGERY

Introduction

The use of imagery to enhance physical and mental health dates back to ancient cultures. Historical data from Assyria, Babylonia, and Greece describe rituals that used imagery to heal diseases in afflicted persons. Furthermore, imagery has long been an important component of Freudian analysis. Currently, guided relaxation imagery is widely used in child psychotherapy. It is a simple, effective, cognitive-behavioral play therapy technique in which a therapist guides a client in imagining a relaxing scene or set of experiences. Numerous clinical observations over the past 30 years have indicated that a person visualizing an imagined scene (e.g., relaxing in a hammock) reacts as if it were actually occurring. Consequently, imagery can have a positive effect on one's physiological and psychological well-being.

Rationale

• The creation of relaxing imagery helps children feel safe and restores feelings of calmness, safety, and well-being when they are experiencing stress and/or upsetting affect, such as anxiety, anger, and sadness. It creates an imaginary "safe place" that can be revisited anytime.

• The ability to imagine calming images promotes a feeling of self-control and well-being and improves functioning.

Description

Ages

Six years and up.

Techniques

The therapist can play a tape that guides a child through a standard relaxing scene or he/she can read a guided relaxation imagery script (available from the Internet). Alternately, the therapist can help a child create his/her own relaxing imagery. One procedure for the latter approach is to explain that you are going to tell how to use one's imagination to help the child feel good when he/she is tense or upset. Then, in a soft voice, ask the child to sit comfortably, take a few deep breaths, close his/her eyes (or look down), and picture in his/her mind a place (real or imaginary) where the child feels very calm, relaxed, and safe. Once the child indicates that he/she has visualized a place, ask him/her to tell you about the safe place. Request that the child include as many sensory details as possible (e.g., what you see, color of the sky; hear, sound of waves breaking; smell, feel, warmth of the sun on your skin; and taste when in the safe place). This intensifies the image and makes it seem more real to the child. After picturing the safe place, ask the child to draw this special place (or do a free drawing just using colors to express the feelings evoked by the mental image). Finally, suggest that the child close his/her eyes and picture this safe, comforting place during times of tension or upset.

Empirical Findings

1. The effectiveness of guided relaxation imagery has been established by research findings that demonstrate its positive impact on physical and psychological well-being. For instance, Ball, Shapiro, Monheim, and Weydert (2003) reported that children with recurrent abdominal pain who received four sessions of relaxation and guided imagery training experienced a 67% decrease in pain. Similarly, Van Tilburg (2009) found that the guided imagery technique significantly reduced functional stomach pain in children.

2. Ebrahim, Elliott, and Summers (1982) reported that after a training program integrating relaxation training and hypnosis, children and adolescents improved their self-concept and gained control of serious behavior problems, such as anorexia nervosa, attention, and poor impulse control.

Applications

The guided relaxation imagery technique has been successfully applied to a wide variety of childhood psychological disorders, including generalized anxiety, stress reactions, fears/phobias, OCD, PTSD, trauma and abuse, depression, ADD/ADHD, habit disorders, and sleep disorders.

Contraindications

Children who dissociate may not be good candidates for this activity.

References

Ball, T., Shapiro, D., Monheim, C., & Weydert, J. (2003). A pilot study of the use of guided imagery for the treatment of recurrent abdominal pain in children. *Clinical Pediatrics*, 42(6), 527–532.
Casement, M., & Swanson, L. (2012). A meta-analysis of imagery rehearsal for post-trauma nightmares. *Clinical Psychology Review*, 32(6), 566–574.

Desoille, R. (1945). *Le reve eveille en psychotherapie.* Paris: Presses Universitaires de France.

Desoille, R. (1961). *Theorie et pratique de reve eveille dirige.* Geneva, Switzerland: Mont Blanc.

Ebrahim, D., Elliott, J., & Summers, J. (1982). The use of hypnosis with children and adolescents. *International Journal of Clinical and Experimental Hypnosis, 30*(2), 189–234.

Gardner, R. (1971). *Therapeutic communication with children: The mutual storytelling technique.* Northvale, NJ: Jason Aronson.

Hackman, A. (2011). Imagery rescripting in posttraumatic stress disorder. *Cognitive and Behavioral Practice, 18,* 424–432.

Halliday, G. (1987). Direct psychological therapies for nightmares: A review. *Clinical Psychology Review, 7,* 501–523.

Hansen, K., Hofling, V., Kroner-Barowik, T., Strangier, U., & Steil, R. (2013). Efficacy of psychological interventions aiming to reduce chronic nightmares: A meta-analysis. *Clinical Psychology Review, 32*(1), 146–155.

Klinger, E. (1980). Therapy and the flow of thought. In J. Shorr, G. Sobel, P. Robin, & J. A. Connella (Eds.), *Imagery: Its many dimensions and application.* New York: Plenum Press.

Krakow, B. (2001). Imagery rehearsal therapy for chronic nightmares: A randomized, controlled trial. *Journal of the American Medical Association, 286,* 537–545.

Oransky, K. G. (2011). *How Zac got his Z's: A guide to getting rid of nightmares.* Creative Space Independent Publishing Platform.

Richardson, A. W. (1969). *Mental imagery.* London: Routledge.

Sherrod, L. R., & Singer, J. L. (1984). The development of make-believe play. In J. H. Goldstein (Ed.), *Sports, games, and play* (pp. 1–38). Hillsdale, NJ: Erlbaum.

Siegel, A. (1998). *Dreamcatching: Every parent's guide to exploring and understanding children's dreams and nightmares.* New York: Random House.

Simard, V., & Nielsen, T. (2009). Adaptation of imagery rehearsal therapy for nightmares in children: A brief report. *Psychotherapy: Theory, Research, Practice, Training, 46*(4), 492–497.

St-Onge, M., Mercier, P., & De Koninck, J. (2009). Imagery rehearsal therapy for frequent nightmares in children. *Behavioral Sleep Medicine, 7*(2), 81–89.

Van Tilburg, M. (2009). Audio-recorded guided imagery treatment reduces abdominal pain in children. *Pediatrics, 124*(5), e890–e897.

37

The World Technique

Introduction

Children delight in playing in the sand, joining their inner and outer worlds together through imaginative play. The world technique was created in 1929 by British pediatrician/child psychiatrist Margaret Lowenfeld (1935) at the Institute of Child Psychology in London. She reported that the idea for the technique came from reading the book *Floor Games* by H. G. Wells (1911). In the book Wells described spending many hours playing on the floor with his two sons. During this play they created fantastic islands with toy soldiers and building blocks. He observed that through this play, his sons worked out problems they had with each other and with other members of the family.

Rationale

Lowenfeld (1979) believed that young children were able to express conscious and unconscious emotions and needs that they were unable to express in words by using concrete, sensory play materials. Once the child's thoughts, feelings, and images were projected and externalized in their sand world, the child was able to gain a greater awareness and insight into his/her life. Indeed, many child therapists have observed that unresolved problems, unfinished tasks, role conflicts, and challenges to identity often emerge in the sand pictures of children (Klinger, 1971). Bringing these issues into personal consciousness is the first step in disempowering them and allowing them to be overcome.

In sum, the main therapeutic powers of the world technique are that it promotes healing by fostering client self-expression, self-awareness, and self-exploration.

Description

Ages

Four years and up.

Materials

Lowenfeld (1979) provided a rectangular tray, about 30 inches long, 20 inches wide, and 4 inches deep, on a table that places the tray at waist height for the child. The tray was half-filled with wet or dry sand. A cabinet with pull-out drawers containing over a hundred miniature figures was nearby for the child to place in the sandtray. According to Lowenfeld, the miniature collection should include all the objects needed to make a small world, including:

- "Living creatures," including men, women, and children, and both wild and domestic animals.
- "Fantasy and folklore" figures, including prehistoric creatures, mythological creatures, and deities.
- "Scenery," including buildings, trees, fences, gates, and bridges.
- "Transport" for road, rail, sea, and air travel.
- "Equipment" for farms, hospitals, and roads (e.g., traffic signs).

Techniques

Lowenfeld's (1950) instruction to the child was, "We have pictures in our heads we can't put into words and its fun sometimes to create something without being concerned if it is realistic or not" (p. 327). Alternately, one might say, "As you can see, this tray is filled with sand. Pick as few or as many of these small toys and build a scene in the sand . . . or anything else that comes to mind. There is no right or wrong way to do this." Typically, the child is given complete freedom to select and arrange the figures in the tray. The role of the therapist is to be a silent witness who is full of wonder as the child creates a sand scene. When the scene is complete, the therapist asks a few questions to help the child more fully understand what has been expressed. As the first therapist to espouse a child-centered orientation, Lowenfeld believed that no interpretations or advice should be offered, so that the child can form his/her own meaning and associations to the sand picture. She believed that there were healing forces within children that enable them to find adaptive solutions to their problems. The therapist provides the key to making this happen by nondirective sandplay (Lanyado & Horne, 1999). Lowenfeld believed that the meaning of symbolic objects in the sand scene are self-evident to the mind that used them. She termed her intervention "direct projection therapy."

The world technique has formed the basis for the development of two popular forms of play therapy. Jungian play therapists (Kalff, 2003) have applied Jung's principles to the world technique in an approach called "sandplay therapy." Jungians are particularly interested in understanding the healing symbols and archetypes represented in the child's sandplay creations. "Sandtray therapy" (Homeyer & Sweeney, 2010) is the name used by therapists who espouse alternate theoretical orientations, such as the humanistic, Adlerian, Gestalt, and prescriptive approaches. At present, there is no evidence that recent therapeutic approaches are more effective than the original world technique. The fact that it has stood the test of time and is so widely utilized is a testament to Lowenfelds' (1950) original insights into the play preferences and therapeutic needs of young children. Many play therapists today report that the one item in the playroom that they could not do without is a sandtray.

Variations

Therapist-Guided Scenes

Following a structured approach, a therapist might ask children to make a scene in the sand that represents their family, or create scenes representing their life before and after their parents' divorce. A therapist might ask adolescents to create a scene depicting their career goals. After the scene is constructed, the therapist would conduct an inquiry to deepen the client's self-awareness and understanding by asking questions such as:

"Where are you in this scene, or where would you like to be in the scene?"
"What would you like to be different about the scene?"
"What is going to happen next in the scene?"
"What would be a good title for the scene?"

Group Sandplay

The therapist gives each member of a child play group a sandtray and a selection of miniatures to play with. Although no specific instruction to build a "world" is given, most children—5 years or older—create a scene in the sand. The group members then take turns sharing with one another their thoughts and feelings about their sand construction.

Family Sandtray

This technique involves asking each member of the family to create a scene in his/her individual sandtray depicting their family doing something together. The therapist asks follow-up questions to clarify each family member's sand creations.

Tabletop World

With preschool children the therapist might simply invite them to play on a table (or floor) with a selection of miniature figures (animals, people, houses, trees, cars, and so forth). The therapist observes any themes that emerge from the play.

Empirical Findings

Flahive and Ray (2007) found that preadolescent clients who participated in group sandtray therapy for 10 weeks showed significant improvement in both externalizing and internalizing behavior problems compared with the wait-list control group.

Applications

The use of sandtrays and miniatures to help clients resolve diverse problems by helping them become aware of their inner world of thoughts and feelings is being widely used by play therapists around the world. Children, adolescents, couples, and the elderly have been found to be receptive to and benefit from this approach.

References

Flahive, M., & Ray, D. (2007). Effect of group sandtray therapy with preadolescents. *Journal for Specialists in Group Work, 32*(4), 362–382.

Homeyer, L., & Sweeney, D. (2010). *Sandtray: A practical manual* (2nd ed.). New York: Routledge.

Kalff, D. (2003). *Sandplay: A psychotherapeutic approach to the psyche.* Cloverdale, CA: Temenous Press.

Klinger, E. (1971). *Structure and function of fantasy.* New York: Wiley.

Lanyado, M., & Horne, A. (1999). *The handbook of child and adolescent psychotherapy.* London: Routledge.

Lowenfeld, M. (1935). *Play in childhood.* London: MacKeith Press.

Lowenfeld, M. (1950). The nature and use of the Lowenfeld world technique in work with children and adults. *Journal of Psychology, 30,* 325–331.

Lowenfeld, M. (1979). *Understanding children's sandplay: Lowenfeld's world technique.* London: Allen & Udwin.

Wells, H. G. (1911). *Floor games.* London: Frank Palmer.

38

Dollhouse Play

Introduction

The earliest recorded construction of a dollhouse was by Albert Duke of Bavaria in 1550. It was a copy of his own residence and he used it to display evidence of his prosperity. Since the beginning of the 20th century, dollhouses have become a classic therapy toy because children find them so enjoyable to play with and they facilitate the expression of a child's view of his/her family life (Klem, 1992; Olszerski & Fuson, 1982).

Virginia Axline (1947, 1964) was among the first play therapists to discuss the effectiveness of the dollhouse as a tool for uncovering the family dynamics of children. Since that time, dollhouse play has become established as a powerful tool for eliciting young children's views of their family life (Woolgar, 1999) and for helping them work through a wide variety of issues and concerns.

Rationale

Typically, young children are better able to express their thoughts and feelings about their home life (e.g., nurturing or hostile) by projecting them in dollhouse play than by trying to state them verbally (Tallandini, 2004).

Description

Ages

Three to 10 years.

Materials

There are countless dollhouses available but only a few are suitable for play therapy. The dollhouse itself should have the following qualities:

- Allow for easy access by having an open top or open side so the figures and objects can be freely moved in and out of the rooms.
- Have an attractive, inviting appearance. The color should be gender neutral to also appeal to young boys.
- Be comfortable to use by being elevated on a low table so it is waist high.
- Be realistic. The rooms and people should correspond to those in the real life of the child. The people should be bendable and able to stand. The house itself should have a contemporary look.
- Be well stocked with family figures and furniture.

Techniques

In addition to giving the child the opportunity to play freely with one or two dollhouses if the child lives in more than one home, a number of structured techniques are useful.

Dollhouse Play Task

Structured doll play assessment was very popular in the 1950s and there has been a strong resurgence of interest in this technique in recent years. In this technique (Murray & Woolgar, 1999), the therapist presents four universal, family-based scenes using a dollhouse and doll materials. The therapist asks the child to show and tell what happens in his/her own family during each of the four scenarios:

1. Bedtime. "Now it's bedtime. Show me what happens in your house at bedtime."
2. Dinnertime.
3. Playtime.
4. Cleanup time.

The therapist listens to each of these scenarios in a reflective, nondirective manner.

A similar procedure was developed by Lynn and Lynn (1959) using 10 scenarios, including toilet time, child afraid of the dark, and siblings fighting over a toy. The following two techniques represent more recent variations of the structured dollhouse play assessment procedure.

Story Stems

This technique involves presenting the child with story starters that the child uses to enact a story using small family dolls and dollhouse furniture. Research has established the connection between these dollhouse stories and the family relationships in the child's actual family life (Warren, Oppenheim, & Emde, 1996). An example of a story stem is "This is a family having dinner and little Jane here just spilled her milk. Show and tell me what happens next." Another story stem might involve a child who just hurt his/her knee, saw a monster in his/her bedroom, encounters a scary dog, or whose mom cancels a play date (Warren, Emde, & Soufe, 2000). The themes that arise in this structured play most often center on mastery and other issues, and conflicts the child has been unable to gain control over (Semrud-Clikeman, 1995).

Daily Events

In this technique, the therapist presents the child with a dollhouse and doll figures representing his/her family and asks the child to show and tell about the daily events at home (Gil, 1994; Tallandini, 2004)—for example, using the dollhouse, the child is asked to show what happens in the family (1) during mealtimes, (2) at bedtime, (3) on the saddest day, and (4) on the happiest day. Play therapists can learn a lot about a child's home life by paying attention to these replays of family events.

Two Houses

Show the child small family dolls and two dollhouses. Then say: "Here are two houses. Let's suppose that this is the house where your family is living now, but because of work being done on the house some members of your family need to live in this other house for a while. Who would you like to go live in this house? Anyone else?" (Kuhli, 1979).

Away-from-Home Scenarios

Apart from home scenarios, a child might be presented with toy props representing a schoolroom, a hospital room, or a courtroom, and asked to show with the miniature toys and people what happens there.

Case Illustrations

- Klem (1992) reported that dollhouse play helped a young boy disclose and process the trauma of physical abuse by his father and older brother. The dollhouse play helped the boy overcome the feelings of helplessness and isolation he felt during the abuse.

- Walker (1989) related the case of a 7-year-old girl who played with a doll family in a dollhouse. She had the father doll put the little girl doll to bed and then the father doll got into the child's bed.

• In Virginia Axline's book *Dibs in Search of Self* (1964), a young boy named Dibs acted out his family problems using a dollhouse. A particularly distressing experience for Dibs was being locked in a room by his parents.

• Marvasti (2004) described the case of Jimmy, who was resentful of the arrival of a baby sister. In his second session, he arranged the family dolls inside the dollhouse. Then he had the mother doll buy a new puppy, which became the center of attention. He then had a monster from outside come in and kidnap the new puppy (symbolic of baby sister).

Empirical Findings

1. Trawick-Smith (1990) found that realistic toy props (e.g., dollhouse family and furniture vs. nonrealistic props—monsters stimulate the greatest amount of pretend play in children under the age of 5 years). The ambiguous features of non-realistic toys tend to lead to exploration of the toy ("What is this object?"), rather than playing imaginatively with the object.

2. Murray and Woolgar (1999) reported that dysfunctional parent–child interactions tend to be reflected in the dollhouse play of children ages 4–8 years.

3. Beiser (1955) gave young children a variety of toys and play materials and observed that they chose to play most often with the dollhouse family. She also noted that children were best able to express feelings about their home situation with doll play.

Applications

Dollhouse play can be an effective window into the home life of all children ages 3–10 years, especially children ages 5–8 years. It is often used for children of divorce or separation and those struggling with conflict between themselves and parents or siblings. It can also facilitate a child's disclosure of physical/sexual abuse, neglect, and domestic violence (Hodges, Hule, & Hillman, 2003; Klem, 1992).

References

Axline, V. (1947). *Play therapy: The inner dynamics of children.* Oxford, UK: Houghton Mifflin.

Axline, V. (1964). *Dibs in search of self.* New York: Houghton Mifflin.

Beiser, H. R. (1955). Play equipment. *American Journal of Orthopsychiatry, 25,* 761–771.

Gil, E. (1994). *Play in family therapy.* New York: Guilford Press.

Hodges, J., Hule, M., & Hillman, S. (2003). Changes in attachment representations over the first year of adoptive placement: Narratives of maltreated children. *Clinical Child Psychology and Psychiatry, 8*(3), 351–367.

Klem, R. (1992). The use of the dollhouse as an effective disclosure technique. *International Journal of Play Therapy*, 1(1), 69–78.

Kuhli, L. (1979). The use of two houses in play therapy. *American Journal of Orthopsychiatry*, 49(3), 431–435.

Lynn, B., & Lynn, R. (1959). The structured doll house play test. *Journal of Projective Techniques*, 23, 335–344.

Marvasti, J. A. (Ed.). (2004). *Psychiatric treatment of victims and survivors of sexual trauma*. Springfield, IL: Charles C. Thomas.

Murray, L., & Woolgar, M. (1999). Children's social representations in dolls' house play and theory of mind tasks and their relation to family adversity and child disturbance. *Social Development*, 8(2), 179–200.

Olszewski, P., & Fuson, K. (1982). Verbally expressed fantasy play of preschoolers as a function of toy structure. *Developmental Psychology*, 18(1), 57–61.

Semrud-Clikeman, M. (1995). *Child and adolescent therapy*. Boston: Allyn & Bacon.

Tallandini, M. (2004). Aggressive behavior in children's dolls' house play. *Aggressive Behavior*, 30, 504–519.

Trawick-Smith, J. (1990). The effects of realistic versus non-realistic play materials on young children' symbolic transformation of objects. *Journal of Research in Childhood Education*, 3(1), 27–36.

Walker, C. (1989). Use of art and play therapy in pediatric oncology. *Journal of Pediatric Oncology*, 6(4), 121–126.

Warren, S., Emde, R., & Soufe, A. (2000). Internal representations predicting anxiety from children's play narratives. *Journal of the American Academy of Child and Adolescent Psychiatry*, 39(1), 100–124.

Warren, S., Oppenheim, D., & Emde, R. (1996). Can emotions and themes in children's play predict behavior problems? *Journal of the American Academy of Child and Adolescent Psychiatry*, 35, 1331–1337.

Woolgar, M. (1999). Projective doll play methodologies for preschool play. *Child Psychology and Psychiatry*, 4(3), 126–134.

39

Adaptive Doll Play

Introduction

Doll play has been a popular form of children's pretend play for decades. By age 3 years children use simple, realistic dolls to act out family roles and situations. Adaptive doll play is a specific doll play technique that involves a therapist or parent using miniature dollhouse dolls and furniture to replicate a stressful situation that the child is experiencing and to model a more adaptive way to handle it.

Rationale

This technique is used to model effective problem solving for children experiencing behavior problems at home. Playing with miniature dolls and objects allows children to work on the problem in a manageable way. According to Bandura (1971), the predominant way young children learn is through observational learning (i.e., observing the behavior of others). This form of learning does not require reinforcement. It simply requires someone or something to model the desired behavior (e.g., a parent, teacher, therapist, peer, or doll).

Description

Ages

Three to 7 years.

Materials

Miniature doll family and dollhouse furniture. A dollhouse may also be used but is not required.

Techniques

This is a directive technique (Brennan, 1990, 2001; Danger, 2003; Lynn & Lynn, 1959) that begins with the therapist or parent setting up a relatable scenario for a story to tell and act out for the child using miniature dolls and dollhouse furniture. The doll representing the child should be of similar age and gender, and have a similar behavior problem as the client. The technique involves a therapist reenacting with a miniature doll family and dollhouse furniture a home situation that is difficult for the child. The therapist uses the props to model a more positive way the child can handle the situation (e.g., parental separation, sleeping alone at night, sharing toys with siblings). For best results, the more adaptive behaviors should be repeated four or five times to solidify the learning. These replays give the child a positive picture that is easier to remember than words.

Empirical Findings

The adaptive doll play technique is in need of empirical research.

Applications

In addition to fostering self-expression in children, this technique can be used to show and tell children a story that models positive ways to cope with common childhood difficulties, such as going to bed or falling asleep, separation anxiety (Danger, 2003), peer conflict resolution (Chittenden, 1942), and parental separation/divorce-related stresses.

References

Bandura, A. (1971). *Psychological modeling.* New York: Lieber-Antheton.

Brennan, C. A. (1990). Parent adaptive doll play with children experiencing parental separation/divorce. *Dissertation Abstracts International, 51,* 4022.

Brennan, C. A. (2001). The parent adaptive doll play technique. In C. E. Schaefer & H. G. Kaduson (Eds.), *101 more favorite play therapy techniques* (pp. 294–298). Northvale, NJ: Jason Aronson.

Chittenden, G. B. (1942). An experimental study in measuring and modifying assertive behavior in young children. *Monograph of the Society for Research in Child Development, 7*(1, Serial No. 31).

Danger, S. (2003). Adaptive doll play: Helping children cope with change. *International Journal of Play Therapy, 12*(1), 105–116.

Lynn, D., & Lynn, R. (1959). The structured doll play test as a projective technique for use with children. *Journal of Projective Techniques, 23*(3), 335–344.

40

Rosebush Fantasy Technique

Introduction

The rosebush fantasy technique is a projective drawing exercise, created by John Stevens in 1971. The technique enables individuals to project feelings, needs, and experiences onto a rosebush; identify with the rosebush; and reown parts of them that had been put out of awareness. This helps individuals reconnect with unpleasant/disconnected experiences and aspects of their lives.

Violet Oaklander (1978, 1997), a Gestalt child therapist, adapted the exercise to help children and adolescents express blocked feelings, thoughts, and needs in a nonthreatening way. The technique is helpful for individuals, families, and groups.

Rationale

This exercise incorporates the use of guided imagery, fantasy, and metaphorical thinking—three therapeutic factors of effective play therapy. Using the metaphor of a rosebush, this exercise provides a way for children to express fears, problems, desires, needs, and thoughts in a safe, disguised manner. In addition, Oaklander (1997) found that children gain a stronger sense of self when they have the opportunity to look at and address aspects of the metaphor that pertain to their lives.

The rosebush fantasy technique offers a number of therapeutic benefits. These include:

• *Communication.* The rosebush technique provides a way for children to express conscious and unconscious wishes, conflicts, fears, and fantasies in a creative and enjoyable manner. This provides therapists with useful information for establishing treatment goals.

• *Concretization.* The rosebush drawing embodies aspects of the child's internal world and emotional life that can be addressed in a disguised manner. It provides play therapists with access to the child's inner world and fosters the therapist's understanding of the child's difficulties and needs.

• *Creative thinking.* The metaphor of a rosebush encourages flexible thinking, the ability to play with new ideas, and increased insight into personal problems and feelings. In addition, thinking of ideas and solutions for the rosebush can help children find solutions to difficulties in their lives.

• *Fantasy.* Oaklander (1997) noted that the use of guided fantasy and imagery inherent in the rosebush techniques helps children express emotions and needs that are blocked. She wrote, "The use of fantasy provides a bridge to the child's inner life. The child then can look at it, examine it, and when ready, own it" (p. 11).

• *Metaphorical thinking.* The metaphor of a rosebush, which represents the child, makes this a powerful therapeutic technique. Understanding the rose imparts an understanding of the child's unconscious feelings and difficulties. Oaklander (1997) contends that the child's self is strengthened when he/she "owns" aspects of the rosebush metaphor that pertain to disconnected aspects of his/her life.

Description

Ages

Ten to 16 years.

Techniques

The rosebush technique involves five steps:

1. Instructing the child to close his/her eyes and imagine that he/she is a rosebush.
2. Asking the child to describe physical and geographic features of the rosebush such as size; shape; whether it has roots, thorns, or flowers; color of flowers; where it is located; what is next to it; and who takes care of it.
3. Asking the child to draw the rosebush and whatever else he/she would like in the pictur.;
4. Asking the child to tell the therapist the story of the rosebush drawing.
5. Asking the child if the characteristics and story about the rosebush pertains to any aspect of the child's life.

Case Illustration

Ray, Perkins, and Oden (2004) administered the rosebush fantasy technique to three fifth-grade students. Their description and interpretation of the students'

drawings demonstrates the utility of the technique for accessing the phenomeno-
logical experience of children. Their description of a child named Roger, a fifth-
grade student identified with an emotional disturbance and speech impairment,
provides a vivid example. They wrote:

> Roger attends his current elementary school because his father has threatened to
> abduct him from his home elementary school. He lives with a cousin and is very aware
> that his father is threatening to abduct him from school. At school, Roger attempts
> to make everyone around him happy. In processing his rosebush, Roger described his
> rosebush as colorful and always tired. In describing his stems and branches he stated,
> "My stems suck up the water so they can live. The branches are connected to the stems
> and the trunk. They were helping me suck water out of the soil." Roger reported that
> he did not have any thorns and that nothing protects him. When the counselor asked
> how it felt to not have thorns, Roger replied, "It doesn't feel good at all. When some-
> thing picks me up, I would die if I didn't have thorns. If I did have thorns, I could hurt
> somebody." Roger further stated that his rosebush is grumpy when he tells others to
> quit what they are doing because it bothers him, but they keep doing it and not listen-
> ing to him. Further, he is happy when he asks somebody to stop it and they listen to
> him. When asked about what he would change about his picture, Roger responded,
> "I would draw two rosebush trees with thorns so that they would protect me. I would
> also add thorns to my rosebush. I wouldn't like living by myself." (pp. 4–5)

Empirical Findings

1. Allan and Crandall (1986) developed the rosebush visualization strategy to
test the validity of the rosebush fantasy technique. In this study, three school counselors used rosebush drawings to distinguish coping from noncoping children with
80% accuracy. The pictures (visual imagery) and the words used to describe the
rosebush (metaphorical statements) by coping children reflected emotional health.
Those of noncoping children showed inner turmoil.

2. Glazer (1998) studied rosebush drawings of bereaved children before and
after they participated in a grief-counseling program. The study found positive
changes in the children's drawings following the grief-counseling program. Specifically, the postcounseling drawings were interpreted as more connected and better
organized.

Applications

The projective nature of the rosebush technique makes it an excellent tool for
children who have difficulty expressing emotions about painful experiences. It
provides depressed and anxious children as well as those with early losses and/or
traumas a way to express feelings and needs in a nonthreatening way. The rosebush
drawing technique can be used with any child who is capable of understanding the

directions and drawing a rosebush. However, Ray et al. (2004) note that young children often have difficulty connecting aspects of the drawing to their real-life situations because doing so requires abstract reasoning that develops later.

References

Allan, J., & Crandall, J. (1986). The rosebush: A visualization strategy. *Elementary School Guidance and Counseling, 21*, 44–51.

Glazer, H. (1998). Expressions of children's grief: A qualitative study. *International Journal of Play Therapy, 7*(2), 51–65.

Oaklander, V. (1978). *Windows to our children: A Gestalt therapy approach to children and adolescents*. Highland, NY: Gestalt Journal Press.

Oaklander, V. (1997). The rosebush. In H. G. Kaduson & C. E. Schaefer (Eds.), *101 favorite play therapy techniques* (pp. 11–13). Northvale, NJ: Jason Aronson.

Ray, D. C., Perkins, S. R., & Oden, K. (2004). Rosebush fantasy technique with elementary school students. *Professional School Counseling, 7*(4), 277–282.

Stevens, J. O. (1971). *Awareness: Exploring, experimenting, expressing*. Moab, UT: Real People Press.

41

Family Relations Technique

Introduction

The family relations technique was initially developed over 50 years ago by Eva Bene, a psychiatrist, and James Anthony, a psychologist, as a projective technique to assess children's views of their family relationships (Bene & Anthony, 1957). It has remained a popular clinical tool ever since.

Rationale

The quality of children's family relationships has a major impact on their sense of self, their development of secure attachments, their self-esteem, and their overall psychological well-being. Often, young children find it difficult to verbally express positive or negative feelings about their family members. Since words are not needed in this technique, it facilitates emotional expression and enhances insight, which can lead to more effective problem solving and improvements in family relations. The use of this technique for initial and ongoing assessment of the child's perception of family members provides a rich source of information for treatment planning.

Description

Ages

Three to 17 years.

Materials

About five to 10 miniature toy mailboxes (commercially available from such sites as Oriental Trading, Target, and Dollar Stores). In addition, about 25–75 small slips of paper are needed to serve as "mail" for the boxes.

Techniques

Place the mailboxes on a table in front of the child, one for each member of the family, including the child, and one labeled "Mr. Nobody" for mail that does not belong to any family member. The mail consists of the small slips of paper with a simple, clear statement that you have written on each describing possible positive and negative beliefs a child this age might have about family members. Examples of statements you might prepare for the child are:

"Loves me."
"Plays with me."
"Hits me."
"Hates me."
"Yells at me."
"I like to cuddle with."
"Teases me."
"Scares me."
"Protects me."
"Spoils me."

Read each note and ask the child to place it in the mailbox of the family member the child feels it best describes. Each mailbox has a card in front with the name of the family member to which it belongs. The postings are reviewed by the therapist to gain a deeper understanding of the child's family relationships and their relevance to the child's presenting problem.

Variations

1. The mailbox procedure can be used to help children send messages to lost or distant loved ones (grief work), to past or future selves, or to send to others about subjects difficult to express directly.

2. Bow (1988) created a procedure entitled the "family word association game." In this game, the child is asked to draw a picture of each member of his/ her family doing something together. Then the therapist gives the child a stack of cards, each containing the name of a positive or negative personal attribute (e.g., pretty, fun, protective, mean, person in charge, gets mad easily, not around much, I'm closest to, cries a lot). The child is asked to place each card on the person it best describes. If the card does not apply to anyone in the family, it is placed in the "Nobody" pile (no more than 10 cards can be placed in this pile). The child may add self-made cards to the premade stack. The card selections are recorded by the therapist and subsequently discussed with the child for a fuller understanding of the child's view of family relationships.

3. Surkin's (2001) variation of the family attribute game asks the child to first complete a KFD and then place colorful index cards (3 × 5 inches) with a specific attribute on it in a pile next to the name of each family member. Both positive and negative personal attributes are included, such as "Saddest," "Most fun to be with," and "Cries a lot." The child is invited to add additional attribute cards of his/her own choosing.

Empirical Findings

The family relations technique is in need of empirical research.

Applications

The family relations technique and variations of it are child-friendly methods that foster self-expression and insight in children. They provide invaluable information for therapists regarding children's thoughts, feelings, and unmet needs as well as family dynamics, alliances, and other issues. The family relations technique can be used with all children but is particularly useful for children with problematic family relations, sibling or parent–child conflict, and issues related to separation or divorce.

References

Bene, E., & Anthony, E. J. (1957). *Manual for the Family Relations Test*. Slough, UK: National Foundation for Educational Research in England and Wales.

Bow, J. (1988). Treating resistant children. *Child and Adolescent Social Work, 5*, 3–15.

Surkin, E. (2001). Variation of the family attribute game. In H. G. Kaduson & C. E. Schaefer (Eds.), *101 more favorite play therapy techniques* (pp. 337–339). Northvale, NJ: Jason Aronson.

42

Worry Dolls

Worry never robs tomorrow of its sorrow,
it only saps today of its joy.
—LEO BUSCAGLIA

Introduction

Worry dolls are miniature handmade dolls dressed in colorful Mayan outfits. Made in Guatemala from wire, cloth, and yarn, Guatemalan worry dolls are usually between ½ inch and 2 inches tall. They often come in cloth pouches or wooden boxes in sets of six to eight. According to Mayan legend, indigenous people have used worry dolls for centuries to relieve their children of worries at bedtime. When a child is unable to sleep, he/she assigns each worry to one of the worry dolls and places them under his/her pillow or in their pouch or box. The dolls take over the worrying for the child, who then sleeps peacefully.

Rationale

Worry dolls are tiny, colorful, and unique. Young children are fascinated by the legend of worry dolls and their appearance makes them fun and engaging. These qualities make worry dolls a useful technique in play therapy for children ages 4 years and up. Their therapeutic benefits include:

• *Therapeutic relationship.* Because worry dolls are engaging, they can be used as an ice-breaker to teach children that everyone (even people in other countries such as Guatemala) has worries. This process frees the child to acknowledge his/her worries in a playful, nonthreatening way and helps the therapist establish rapport and trust.

• *Communication.* Worry dolls foster the expression and sharing of worries and other negative feelings—for example, when used for children of cancer survivors (U.C. Davis Health System, n.d.), worry dolls were described as "special friends" with whom they could share emotional pain. In addition, one of the children stated "that she didn't need to tell the worry doll her worries anymore, because the doll just knows them now."

• *Mastery.* Children often become engrossed in the process of making worry dolls. This process gives them a sense of competence, efficacy, and mastery over unwanted feelings and serves to reduce anxiety and foster self-esteem. Gettins (2014) recommends worry dolls for group work with children exposed to domestic violence. She uses worry dolls with the book *The Huge Bag of Worries* (Ironside, 2012) to teach children the importance of getting worries out, exploring emotions, sharing experiences, and developing coping strategies.

• *Externalization.* Worry dolls provide an object on which children can put their worries. This frees children from anxiety. When children make their own worry dolls they can be brought home and used whenever anxiety occurs; while studying for tests, when separations are impending; and as part of a bedtime ritual. In the latter, parents may take the doll away during the night to reinforce the child's belief that the worry is gone. A container, box, or pouch is helpful to strengthen the child's belief that worries are put away.

Description

Ages

Four years and up.

Materials

Set of Guatemalan worry dolls.

Techniques

During a play therapy session, talk with the child about the worries that he/she would like to be rid of. Then ask the child to assign each worry to a worry doll. Ask the child to put the dolls in their box or pouch and leave them in the office for the week. The dolls can be brought out one by one in subsequent sessions for a discussion about how to resolve them. Authentic Guatemalan worry dolls can be used or children can create personalized worry dolls with a variety of materials. These can include pipe cleaners, yarn, cloth, clothespins, clay, Play-Doh, card stock, and colored markers. Older children, adolescents, or individuals uninterested in "dolls" may prefer to share their worries using stones, beads, marbles, tokens, hearts, or individually crafted objects that can be made with the materials listed above.

Variations

Worry Wall

Like worry dolls, the worry wall technique helps children to externalize their worries. In this technique, children write down or draw a picture of a worry and stick it to the worry wall. Big worries are placed toward the top of the wall and smaller worries toward the bottom. Children then move their worries from session to session, depending on how much the worry affects them (Pomeroy & Garcia, 2009). The therapist might suggest that each worry needs a positive thought to replace it. The child then creates another wall: the optimism wall. The child places two positive thoughts on the optimism wall for each worry on the worry wall.

Worry Can

In this technique (Jones, 1997), children draw or write "scary things" on a piece of construction paper and glue the paper onto a can with a lid. They then make a slot in the top of the lid, and insert small pieces of paper with words or pictures of their worries. A tissue or shoe box decorated as a "worry box" can serve the same purpose. The therapist and child then discuss strategies for resolving the worries.

Worry Stones

This activity, for children ages 3–12 years, can be used with individual children, groups, and families. The therapist and child sit around a large neutral-colored paper that has been placed in the center of the room. Along the wall, stones are placed in three piles: small, medium, and large. The therapist explains that they are worry stones and highlights that sharing worries makes them smaller. Children then select as many stones as needed, to convey the amount and size of their worries. They place their stones on the paper. The therapist starts the game by sharing a worry and the child then has a turn. The game continues until all stones are discussed (Anastasia, 2003).

Worry Time

This focused worry time technique for older children and adolescents involves three steps. First, set aside a specific time, place, and length of time (e.g., 15–20 minutes) for worrying. This should be the same time during the day and not close to bedtime. Next, postpone worrying until the worry time by writing worries down on a notepad you carry with you. Finally, reflect on your worries at the designed worry time.

Anger Expression

A variation for children who have difficulty controlling their anger is to ask them to write down things that make them angry that they would like to let go. The act of writing or drawing about them can help them in identifying and releasing anger in a safer way.

Empirical Findings

Eisenberger, Lieberman, and Williams (2003) showed that putting problems into words eases emotional pain. Using functional magnetic resonance imaging (fMRI), these researchers scanned the brains of individuals as they played a virtual ball-tossing game called "cyberball." The researchers then induced experiences of being excluded/social rejection via a computer program. Social rejection activated the anterior cingulated cortex—a region of the brain that also lights up in response to physical pain. Participants who had less activity in the anterior cingulate cortex and reported feeling less distress, showed more activity in the area of the brain associated with language production and verbalizing thoughts (the right ventral lateral prefrontal cortex). The authors concluded that verbalizing emotions activates the prefrontal cortex, which serves to suppress the region of the brain associated with emotional pain.

Applications

Worry dolls are particularly helpful for overanxious and fearful children, as well for children struggling with insomnia due to anxious thoughts. They have been found to be helpful prompts for discussion of any kind of worry, problem, or negative emotion and can be used for individual, group, or family counseling. We often use worry dolls as an ending ritual to a therapy session. By instructing children to "leave their worries with the worry dolls," they have an opportunity to communicate any concerns they may not have shared during the session. This often reveals valuable information for subsequent sessions and treatment planning. Parents also report that anxious children are "lighter" upon leaving the playroom.

References

Anastasia, J. (2003). Worry stones. In H. G. Kaduson & C. E. Schaefer (Eds.), *101 favorite play therapy techniques* (Vol. 3, pp. 373–378). Lanham, MD: Jason Aronson.

Eisenberger, N. I., Lieberman, M. D., & Williams, K. D. (2003). Does rejection hurt?: A study of social exclusion. *Science, 302*, 290–292.

Gettins, T. (2014). Therapeutic play as an intervention for children exposed to domestic violence. In E. Prendiville & J. Howard (Eds.), *Play therapy today: Contemporary practice with individuals, groups and careers* (pp. 64–78). London: Routledge.

Ironside, V. (2012). *The huge bag of worries*. London: Hachette.

Jones, D. S. (1997). The worry can technique. In H. G. Kaduson & C. E. Schaefer (Eds.), *101 favorite play therapy techniques* (pp. 254–256). Northvale, NJ: Jason Aronson.

Pomeroy, E., & Garcia, R. (2009). *The grief assessment and intervention workbook: A strengths perspective (death and dying/grief and loss)*. Belmont, CA: Brooks/Cole.

U.C. Davis Health System. (n.d.). Worry dolls, posters, masks, and mandalas help kids cope with cancer. Retrieved from *www.ucdmc.ucdavis.edu/welcome/features/20080716_cancer_coping*.

43

Tea Party Play

Introduction

Tea parties are exciting for young children. In real life, parties are a way for people to come together to celebrate holidays, birthdays, milestones, and accomplishments. In the pretend world of play, however, they can take place anytime and for any reason. Pretend play parties are enjoyable for both child and therapist and they foster communication and interpersonal closeness.

Rationale

Tea parties have many therapeutic benefits, including:

- Tea parties help therapists develop rapport with the child in the early stage of play therapy.
- Tea parties make children child feel special and important, which bolsters their self-esteem.
- Tea parties provide a way for a child to learn and practice important social skills, such as sharing, taking turns, initiating conversation, listening to others, and good manners.
- Tea parties create a sense of nurturance in the playroom.

Description

Ages

Four to 8 years.

Materials

Tea party play set (child-size plastic teacups, saucer, plates, and teapot), water, healthy snack, child-size table and chairs.

Techniques

"Tea party" is a classic game that children have played for years. For a tea party the therapist asks the child which guests he/she would like to invite to his/her tea party (e.g., parent, sibling, friend). The child then is asked to pick from home or the play therapy room a doll, plush animal, or puppet to represent each invitee, and place them around the party table. The therapist asks the child to introduce the guests and say something special about them. The party then begins, with the therapist and child taking turns pouring the beverage from the teapot, sharing a snack, and talking with and for the invited guests.

Variation

Celebration Party

The therapist can recognize and reinforce a child's progress in play therapy by surprising the child with a party to celebrate the child's achievement of a therapeutic goal. Party hats, napkins, favors, and treats add to the festivity. On successful termination of the child's therapy, another party is in order.

Empirical Findings

Tea party play is in need of empirical research.

Applications

Tea parties are an excellent way to engage children in treatment and to help them feel welcome and comfortable at the start of therapy. A party is especially helpful to establish rapport with children who are reluctant or resistant to coming to therapy. Celebration parties are helpful for reinforcing children's accomplishments in treatment and to foster motivation for reaching additional treatment goals.

Part Six

GAME PLAY TECHNIQUES

44

Communication Games

> You can discover more about a person in an hour of play than in a year of conversation.
>
> —PLATO

Introduction

A game is an interactional activity of a competitive or cooperative nature involving one or more players who play by a set of rules that define the content of the game (Denzen, 1975). A board game is a game that involves pieces moved or placed on a board according to a set of rules. Board games have been played in most cultures throughout history; some even predate literacy skills in the earliest civilizations. Over the past 30 years, there has been a marked increase in the development of board games for use in psychotherapy with children. There are therapeutic board games designed to enhance a child's self-esteem, self-control, stress management, communication skills, and understanding of a wide variety of childhood problems (e.g., divorce, death, bullying).

Communication board games are designed to enable children to reveal aspects of self, both known and unknown. Often these projections involve the presenting problem as well as additional areas of concern that were not the therapist's initial focus. This gives the therapist a wealth of information about the child. Communication games have been found useful in individual, family, and group therapy.

Rationale

The principle therapeutic benefit of communication games is that they facilitate self-expression by the players. The pretend, "as if" quality of games and the fun and enjoyment derived from playing tend to create a nonthreatening atmosphere and have a "tongue-loosening" effect on children and adolescents. Moreover, the impersonal nature of responding to questions printed on game cards gives players of all ages enough psychological distance to enable them to disclose deep-seated thoughts and feelings. This disclosure serves as a point of departure for subsequent therapeutic discussions with the therapist (Schaefer & Reid, 2001). Among the types of communication elicited through game play are the expression of fantasy and unconscious material, and the disclosure of conscious feelings, thoughts, and wishes.

Description

Ages

Six years and up.

Techniques

Talking, Feeling, Doing Game

The first published therapeutic communication game—The Talking, Feeling, and Doing Game—was created by child psychiatrist Richard Gardner (1973, 2001). It is still one of the most popular tools used by child therapists to facilitate self-expression by children in treatment. This classic game provides enough psychological distance for children to feel free to reveal their underlying thoughts and feelings.

The game cards ask players to answer something regarding a thought, feeling, or action. For example, a "talking" card might say, "Make believe that something is happening that is scary. What is happening?" If players do as the card says, they get a chip. The object of the game is to accumulate as many reward chips as possible. The therapist's responses to the card questions can help correct maladaptive responses of the child.

The Talking, Feeling, and Doing Game has proven developmentally appropriate and useful with school-age children, ages 6–12 years, as an ice-breaker in the early sessions, and as a way to engage even the most resistant and inhibited children to open up and reveal their thoughts and feelings (Fried, 1992).

The Ungame

The Ungame, created by Rhea Zakich (1979), is the world's most popular communication game with over 4 million copies sold (*www.Rheazakich.com*). The game fosters the development of a variety of communications skills, including active listening, expressing your thoughts and feelings clearly, taking turns, understanding others' thoughts and feelings, and remaining quiet while others are speaking.

The game dates back to 1972 when Rhea Zakich, a young mother from Garden City, California, was forced to avoid speaking for months after her doctor discovered polyps on her vocal cords. Although she made a full recovery, the experience of being unable to speak for a long time made her feel emotionally estranged from her husband and two school-age sons. She realized that although they now talked together, they did not really communicate. As a remedy, she decided to write down on paper cards a number of questions that she wanted to ask her family. Some were light-hearted: "What do you like to do in your spare time?"; some serious and intimate: "If you could live your life over, what would you change?"; "What do you think life will be 100 years from now?"; and "What are the four most important things in your life?; "What is your most prized possession?"; What do you wish you had more of from your parents?"

The variations of this popular game include a full game board for all ages, and pocket versions of the cards for children ages 5–12 years, teens, couples, families, and seniors. Therapists use it as an ice-breaker in the first session, or for a serious exchange of thoughts, feelings, and values by family members.

Empirical Findings

The communication games technique is in need of empirical research.

Applications

Communication board games are a highly effective way to facilitate and accelerate self-disclosure by children, adolescents, and adult clients. They also foster the establishment of rapport in individual therapy and cohesion/bonding in group and family therapy.

References

Denzen, N. (1975). Play, games, and interaction. *Sociological Quarterly*, *16*, 468–478.
Fried, S. (1992). Chess: A psychoanalytic tool in the treatment of children. *International Journal of Play Therapy*, *1*, 43–51.
Gardner, R. A. (1973). *The talking, feeling, and doing game.* Cresskill, NJ: Creative Therapeutics.
Gardner, R. A. (2001). The taking, feeling, and doing game. In C. E. Schaefer & S. Reid (Eds.), *Game play: Therapeutic use of childhood games* (2nd ed., pp. 78–105). New York: Wiley.
Schaefer, C. E., & Reid, S. (2001). *Game play: Therapeutic use of childhood games* (2nd ed.). New York: Wiley.
Zakich, R. (1979). *Everybody wins: The story behind the ungame.* Carol Stream, IL: Tyndale House.

45

Self-Control Games

He who controls others may be powerful, but he who has mastered
himself is mightier still.

—LAO TZU

Introduction

Many games have been developed to promote self-control and to improve executive functioning. Executive functioning includes such abilities as *behavioral inhibition*: not acting on impulse; *planning ahead*: anticipating the future, setting goals to guide one's actions; and *working memory*: keeping information in mind so as to complete a task or activity (Yeager & Yeager, 2009). A description of several of these simple and familiar games follows.

Rationale

Children can strengthen their executive functioning ability by deliberately and repeatedly inhibiting their impulsive responses and physical movements over a period of time.

Description

Ages

Three to 12 years.

Techniques

Simon Says

The Simon Says game has been popular with children throughout the world since Roman times. In this game, children follow the directions of the game leader *only* if they are preceded by the leader saying, "Simon says . . . " A command starting with "Simon says" means the players must obey that command. A command *without* the beginning "Simon says" means *do not* obey the command. Players who do not follow the commands are eliminated from the remainder of the game—for example, the leader may say, "Simon says touch your toes!"; "Simon says arms up!"; "Simon says arms down!"; "Arms up!" The latter command must not be obeyed.

The rationale for this game is that it reinforces attention, memory, inhibiting one's impulse to action, and managing frustration. Psychological research has found that self-regulation games, such as Simon Says, are a simple and effective way to help children, ages 8–12 years, improve self-control and restraint of impulsive behavior (Strommen, 1973).

A game similar to Simon Says called Head to Toes requires young children to do the opposite of the instructed command (e.g., to touch their toes when instructed to touch their head, touch their knees when told to touch their shoulders). This self-regulation game requires a combination of attention, inhibition, and memory skills, and has been found to increase self-regulation in preschoolers (Ponitz & McClelland, 2008).

Red Light, Green Light

A game that is also similar to Simon Says is Red Light, Green Light. In this game, children walk or run forward whenever the leader says (or holds up a sign) "Green light" and freeze when they hear "Red light!" This self-control game is particularly appropriate for children with ADHD and impulse-control problems. Tominey and McClelland (2011) reported that the Red Light, Purple Light game improved self-regulation in preschool children who were weak in this skill. The Red Light, Purple Light game follows the same concept as Red Light, Green Light. However, in this game the leader assigns "Go" and "Stop" to nonsequential colors, such as purple and orange.

Statue Game

One person is "it" and the other players move around freely until told to "freeze" like statues. The person who is "it" walks up to each player in turn, and tries without touching the person, to make him/her smile or laugh (e.g., by silly faces, strange noises). The first person to laugh is the next player to be "it" (VanFleet, 2001).

A variation is to play music and when the music stops all the children in the group have to freeze in place. Another variation is to have a child stand motionless like a sentry or ask all the children in a group to lie on the floor and remain quiet and still. If they move they are out. The last child to move is the winner.

Slow Motion Game

With a stopwatch, time a child doing something as slowly as he/she can (e.g., writing his/her full name). The rules are that the child's pencil must always be on the paper and it needs to keep moving all the time. The goal is to break one's previous record for slowness.

Jenga

Jenga is a great game for children with ADHD to play. It requires them to slow down and focus in order to pull a block out without knocking the entire tower of blocks down. It also provides an opportunity for the therapist to discuss how to handle disappointment or frustration when things do not go your way (i.e., the tower falls).

Operation

Operation is a board game that was created over 50 years ago as a game of fine motor skill and self-control. It consists of an "operating table" with a comic likeness of a patient who has a large red lightbulb for his nose. The game requires the player to remove fictional ailments made of plastic with a pair of tweezers without touching the edge of the cavity openings. Touching an opening lights up the red nose and activates a buzzer.

Empirical Findings

1. Halperin, Marks, Bedard, and Chacko (2013) reported that when parents of preschoolers with ADHD were taught to play self-control games (e.g., Simon Says) with their children for at least 30–45 minutes per day over an 8-week period, the children showed significant improvement in ADHD severity, which continued 3 months later.

2. Manuilenko (1948) found that children, ages 3–7 years, "standing sentry" in a room with playmates, managed to stand motionless for significantly longer periods than when they were on their own. This appeared to be result of the playmates "monitoring" the sentry's performance.

Applications

Preschool and school-age children with impulse control problems benefit from self-control games because they teach skills in an enjoyable manner. These games are particularly helpful for children with ADHD and anger control problems.

Children with impulse control problems often require external cues to develop executive functioning before they develop the ability to self-regulate. Training parents of children with impulse control issues to play self-control games at home serves to strengthen executive functioning, improves self-esteem, and fosters closeness between parent and child.

References

Halperin, J., Marks, D., Bedard, A., & Chacko, A. (2013). Training executive, attention, and motor skills: A proof-of-concept study in preschool children with ADHD. *Journal of Attention Disorders*, *17*(8), 711–721.

Manuilenko, Z. (1948). The development of voluntary behavior in preschoolers. *Izvestiya APN RSFSR*, *14*, 43–51.

Ponitz, C., & McClelland, M. (2008). Touch your toes!: Developing a direct measure of behavioral regulation in early childhood. *Early Childhood Research Quarterly*, *23*(2), 141–158.

Strommen, E. (1973). Verbal self-regulation in a children's game: Impulse errors on "Simon Says." *Child Development*, *44*, 849–853.

Tominey, S., & McClelland, M. (2011). Red light, purple light: Findings from a randomized trial using circle time games to improve behavioral self-regulation in preschool. *Early Education and Development*, *22*(30), 489–519.

VanFleet, R. (2001). Make me laugh. In H. G. Kaduson & C. E. Schaefer (Eds.), *101 more favorite play therapy techniques* (pp. 203–206). Northvale, NJ: Jason Aronson.

Yeager, D., & Yeager, M. (2009). *Simon says pay attention* (2nd ed.). Lafayette, LA: Golden Path Games.

46

Strategy Games

> However beautiful the strategy, you should occasionally look
> at the results.
> —WINSTON CHURCHILL

Introduction

Strategy games have specific rules and guidelines for winning and losing and
require skills in planning and problem solving. The challenge and enjoyment that
they offer have made them a source of entertainment in cultures throughout the
world for thousands of years. Ancient Egyptians played the two-person game Senet
as early as 3100 B.C.E. Senet, which means "game of passing," consists of a grid
of 30 squares laid out in three rows of 10. Several squares have symbols on them
representing spiritual and religious themes. The rules used by ancient Egyptians
are unknown. However, historians believe that playing involved both luck and
strategy. Players used sticks or knucklebones as dice to move their pawn around
the board. The first player to remove all pawns was the winner. Imagery found on
ancient tomb walls and on Senet artifacts suggest that ancient Egyptians believed
that winning the game provided spiritual protection. They frequently placed Senet
boards in their tombs in preparation for the afterlife.

Archaeologists have also found evidence of strategy games in China, India,
and Mesopotamia but it wasn't until the Roman conquest that strategy games
emerged in Europe. Popular games among the Romans included (1) Tabula, a
game similar to Backgammon; (2) Calculi, a game similar to Four in a Row; (3)
Latrunculi, a game of military tactics similar to Chess; and (4) Lapilli, a game
similar to Tic-Tac-Toe. The competitive quality of these games reflects the culture
in which they were played, and influenced the development of modern competitive games.

Rationale

Children begin playing board and card games at approximately ages 5–6 years when they acquire logical thinking, problem solving, and an interest in understanding the world. Games provide an easy way for adults to spend unhurried time with children, a factor that nurtures relationships and raises self-esteem. In addition, games foster social, emotional, and cognitive development. Strategy games are especially helpful for teaching children to stop and think, plan ahead, anticipate consequences of actions, control impulses, follow rules, tolerate frustration, and cope with disappointment. In addition, playing a simple strategy game can help play therapists assess a child's ability to stay seated, wait his/her turn, follow rules, pay attention, sustain attention, and handle winning or losing.

Strategy games offer a number of therapeutic benefits. These include:

• *Therapeutic alliance.* Many children enter therapy feeling resistant and/or uncomfortable. The pleasure of playing a familiar game with the therapist can ease these feelings and help the child become engaged in treatment.

• *Mood enhancement.* Game play involves a process of give-and-take that imparts a sense of pleasure and enjoyment. This elevates mood, esteem, and self-worth, and teaches children about the importance of reciprocity.

• *Increased focus and self-discipline.* Strategy games provide a nonthreatening and enjoyable way for children to develop executive functions such as attention, concentration, problem solving, memory skills, anticipation, logical thinking, and frustration tolerance.

• *Socialization.* Children in treatment often have difficulties getting along with others and negotiating social situations. Game play with an empathic therapist teaches sportsmanship and cooperation and helps children to internalize socially acceptable ways to deal with aggression, competition, rules, and boundaries.

• *Mastery.* Freud proposed that game play provides a way for children to express impulses and master anxiety. Game play enables children to master new skills, and fosters the development of executive functions, higher-order thinking, social skills, and a sense of competence and esteem.

• *Healthy competition.* Gardner (2002) notes that competition is beneficial because it allows children to assess their competence by measuring it against the abilities of others. This process fosters confidence and self-esteem. In addition, playing competitive games helps children develop a sense of healthy competition that involves respect for the opponent, winning in a fair and friendly manner, and losing graciously.

Description

Ages

Six years and up.

Techniques

Chess

Historians believe that Chess evolved from a game called Chaturanga or Four Divisions of the Military, which was played in India in 600 C.E. However, it was not until the 15th century that modern Chess became popular in Europe. Chess is a two-person intellectual game that requires concentration, planning, and anticipation. It is commonly used with older children. The board (8 × 8 inches) consists of alternating colors. Each player has 16 pieces that have a different value based on their freedom to move and capture the opponent's pieces. The objective of Chess is to checkmate, or capture the opponent's king.

Often called the founder of Chess therapy, Rhazes, a ninth-century Persian physician, was the first to document the use of Chess as a therapeutic modality. Rhazes used the strategies of the game to help patients understand and master life problems. Since that time, Chess has been used for treating individuals with trust issues, social skills deficits, developmental/spectrum disorders, difficulties speaking about personal problems, impulsivity, poor concentration, and low self-esteem.

Because Chess can be difficult to master, several games have been designed to teach children to play—for example, Chess Teacher by Cardinal Industries is for children ages 6 years and up. Chess pieces are marked with arrows to teach the player what direction the Chess piece can move. No Stress Chess by Winning Moves Games, Inc., is for children ages 7–12 years and includes a deck of action cards. Each card shows a Chess piece and the moves it can make.

Checkers

Historians believe that Checkers, also known as Draughts, originated in the Middle East from a game called Alquerque. Like Chess, Checkers is a two-person game played on a board (8 × 8 inches). However, it is easier to learn and can be played by most children ages 6 years and up. One player has red pieces (often called "men") and the other has black pieces. Players take turns moving their pieces diagonally from one square to another. The goal is to jump over the opponent's pieces and remove them from the board. The first person to capture all the opponent's pieces is the winner. To win the game, players can use an offensive strategy such as jumping the opponent's pieces quickly, a defensive strategy such as positioning pieces to block the opponent, or a combination of both. Also, it is advisable to move pieces forward and to the center because it increases the chance of winning.

Connect Four (Wexler & Strongin, 1974)

First introduced by Milton Bradley in 1974, the game is played with a standing grid (7 × 6 inches). Connect Four is a two-player game for children ages 6 years and up. The objective of the game is to get four counters next to each other in a horizontal, vertical, or diagonal line before the opponent. The game is also called Four in a Row and Captain's Mistress, because it is believed that the game originated by Captain Cook, who played the game alone in his chambers.

UNO

This game was developed by Merle Robbins in 1971 and has been sold by Mattel since 1992. This is a two- to 10-player card game for children ages 7 years and up. The object of the game is to be the first player or team to score 500 points by getting rid of all the cards in his/her hand before the opponent(s). Players do this by matching the card in the discard pile by either number, color, or word. If the player does not have a match, he/she must pick a card from the draw pile. When a player has one card left, he/she must say "Uno!" The hand is over when one player has no cards left. To win the game, players can use an offensive strategy, such as using wild cards to get out of the game, a defensive strategy such as getting rid of high-point cards, or a combination of both.

Pick-Up Sticks

Pick-Up-Sticks were originally made of ivory or bone and historians believe that the game originated in China. However, when it became popular in Colonial America, wood was used to make the sticks and the game was often called Jackstraws or Spellicans. Modern-day Pick-Up-Sticks are usually plastic or wood and are color coded for scoring purposes. Pick-Up-Sticks is a skill game for two or more players ages 5 years and up. Playing requires a flat surface where 30 sticks are dropped into a pile. Players take turns trying to remove a single stick without disturbing the others. If the player succeeds, he/she gets another turn, but if another stick moves, the next player tries. The score is tallied by counting the number of sticks each player picks up, or using the color of the sticks to determine their point value.

Junior Labyrinth (Kobbert, 1995)

Developed by Ravensburger in 1995, this is challenging maze game for one to four players, ages 5 years and up. Players use cute ghosts as playing pieces to move the walls of a castle in search of treasures. The player who collects the most treasure wins.

Empirical Findings

1. Dubow, Huesmann, and Eron (1987) compared the effectiveness of two, 10 session interventions (play therapy vs. cognitive-behavioral therapy) designed to decrease high levels of aggression in 104 boys, ages 8–13 years attending inner-city public schools. Both interventions resulted in significant improvement by decreasing aggression and improving prosocial behaviors immediately following the intervention. However, at a 6-month follow-up, the investigators reported an unexpected finding—namely, only those children who received the play intervention remained significantly improved. The play intervention consisted of dyadic peer play with board and card games. The therapist used modeling, coaching, role play, feedback, and discussion to teach the boys effective strategies to be successful at winning the games. No specific cognitive or behavioral procedure was used. The authors concluded that results might be due to the fact that the boys received a real-life, immediate pay-off for practicing effective strategies such as thinking ahead and considering the consequences of different moves, taking account of their opponent's strategies, and inducing peers to follow rules and await their turn. Elementary school is a time when game play skills are highly valued by the peer group.

2. Serok and Blum (1983) reported that juvenile delinquents had difficulty conforming to the rules during game play and were prone to play aggressively. The delinquents preferred games of chance rather than playing by the rules of strategy games.

3. Unterrainer, Kaller, Halsband, and Rahm (2006) compared how Chess players and non-Chess players of equal intelligence worked on a planning task called the "Tower of London." The findings of this study demonstrated that Chess players spent more time planning their approach and had better-developed planning skills.

4. Levy (1987) reported that playing Chess for at least 1 year promoted self-esteem and improved self-images in perceptually impaired students.

5. Korenman, Tamara, and Lyutykh (2009) found that adolescents who exhibited self-centered and aggressive behaviors were more willing to change their behaviors in a positive way after participating in a school-based Chess program.

Applications

Strategy games are invaluable tools for treating children with aggression, ADHD, impulse control problems, delinquency, social skills difficulties, spectrum disorders, and low self-esteem. They are also very helpful for establishing a therapeutic alliance because they are enjoyable, nonthreatening, and familiar to most children.

References

Cardinal Industries. (2010). *Chess teacher*. Long Island City, NY: Author.

Dubow, E. F., Huesmann, R., & Eron, L. D. (1987). Mitigating aggression and promoting prosocial behavior in aggressive elementary schoolboys. *Behavior Research and Therapy*, *25*(6), 527–531.

Gardner, R. A. (2002). Checkers. In C. E. Schaefer & D. M. Cangelosi (Eds.), *Play therapy techniques* (2nd ed., pp. 329–345). Northvale, NJ: Jason Aronson.

Kobbert, M. (1995). Junior labyrinth [Board game]. Germany: Ravensburg.

Korenman, M., Tamara K., & Lyutykh, E. (2009). Checkmate: A chess program for African-American male adolescents. *International Journal of Multicultural Education*, *11*(1), 1–14.

Levy, W. (1987). Utilizing chess to promote self-esteem in perceptually impaired students: A governor's teacher grant program through the New Jersey State Department of Education.

Robbins, M. (1992). *Uno*. El Segundo, CA: Mattel.

Serok, S., & Blum, A. (1983). Therapeutic use of games. *Residential Group Care and Treatment*, *1*(3), 3–14.

Unterrainer, J. M., Kaller, C. P., Halsband, U., & Rahm, B. (2006). Planning abilities and chess: A comparison of chess and non-chess players on the tower of London task. *British Journal of Psychology*, *97*(3), 299–311.

Wexler, H., & Strongin, N. (1974). Connect four [Board game]. Springfield, MA: Milton Bradley.

47

Cooperative Games

The only thing that will redeem mankind is cooperation.
—BERTRAND RUSSELL

Introduction

Parents and teachers have used cooperative games for many years. During the 1980s companies such as Family Pastimes began manufacturing cooperative board games. These strategy games require that players work together as a team to meet a specific challenge. Players share ideas and strategies, make group decisions, and practice problem solving to obtain a common goal and win the game. This involves listening, sharing, negotiating, and combining forces. Unlike noncompetitive games that focus on playing for enjoyment and have no winner, cooperative games nurture the idea of winning. However, instead of competing against each other, players compete against the game. Because the team either wins together or loses together, cooperative games facilitate caring and appreciation for one another. Children learn that cooperation is not just beneficial for achieving goals but it is also enjoyable and makes them feel valued.

Rationale

Cooperative games teach many skills and have a variety of therapeutic benefits. These include:

- *Relationship enhancement*. Cooperative games are especially helpful for establishing a therapeutic alliance with children. Working together to win a game builds trust and fosters a sense of interpersonal closeness.

220

• *Metaphorical teaching.* Cooperative games are an excellent tool for showing children that therapy is a team approach where the child and therapist work together for a common goal.

• *Social skills.* Cooperative games teach social skills because they require cooperation, sharing, compromise, teamwork, and negotiating in a fun and engaging way.

Description

Ages

Four years and up.

Materials

A variety of cooperative board games are available from *www.familypastimes. com* and *www.drtoy.com.*

Techniques

Max the Cat (Deacove, 1986)

Made by Family Pastimes, this board game is for one to eight players, ages 4–7 years. Players work together to help a mouse, bird, and chipmunk get home safely before Max, the Tomcat, catches them. This game teaches logic, decision making, and cooperative problem-solving skills. It also provides an opportunity for children to express feelings about the fact that Max is a natural hunter.

Mountaineering (Deacove, 1992)

In this game made by Family Pastimes, two to six players, ages 7 years and up, work as a team to reach the summit of a mountain. They share equipment, plan their strategies, and handle obstacles such as frostbite, snow slides, and snow blindness together.

Save the Whales (Kolsbun & Kolsbun, 1978)

This game, made by Animal Town Game Company, is designed for two to four players, ages 8 years and up. Players work together to beat forces such as oil spills and catcher ships that endanger great whales. They win the game when they save eight whales.

Sleeping Grump (Deacove, 1981)

This is a story adventure game, made by Family Pastimes for two to four players, ages 4–7 years. The grump has taken treasures from the villagers. While the grump is fast asleep, players work together to climb to the top of a beanstalk to recover the treasures. However, if the grump is woken up, he takes everything back. Players share the treasures and leave some behind for the grump. Their kindness helps to make him less grumpy. The game is won when everyone has some of the treasure.

Caves and Claws (Deacove, 1998)

This is a fantasy adventure game by Family Pastimes for two to four players, ages 6 years and up. The players work together as a team of archaeologists to head into the jungle to find ancient artifacts. They must overcome obstacles while attempting to create paths, search for treasures, and return alive.

Lord of the Rings (Knizia, 2000)

Based on the fantasy trilogy *Lord of the Rings* by J. R. R. Tolkien (1963), this board game immerses two to five players, ages 12 years and up, into Middle-Earth. Players take on the roles of hobbits and must work together on a quest to destroy the One Ring.

Empirical Findings

1. Deutsch (1949) was among the first researcher to demonstrate experimentally that cooperative learning structures result in greater harmony among people than do competitive games learning structures.

2. Orlick (1981) found that kindergarten children who participated in an 18-week cooperative game program increased their sharing significantly more than did children in a traditional games program.

3. Bay-Hinitz, Peterson, and Quilitch (1994) found that cooperative board game play in children ages 4–5 years significantly decreased aggression and increased cooperative behavior as compared with competitive game play.

4. Garaigordobil, Maganio, and Etxeberria (1996) implemented a 22-session, cooperative game play program for 125 children, ages 6–7 years. Compared with a control group, the children in the intervention group demonstrated positive changes in socioaffective relations and group cooperation. The 54 games were activity and fantasy games rather than board games—for example, groups would build a clay object together, tell a story together, complete a jigsaw puzzle together, or finger paint together.

5. Mender, Kerr, and Orlick (1982) reported that elementary school boys who were involved in a cooperative game program demonstrated a significantly greater increase in cooperative social behaviors than boys who participated in a traditional games program.

Applications

Cooperative games are especially helpful for children who are socially isolated or rejected because of aggressiveness, anxiety/shyness, bossiness, low or inflated self-esteem, or a lack of social skills.

References

Bay-Hinitz, A., Peterson, R. F., & Quilitch, H. (1994). Cooperative games: A way to modify aggressive and cooperative behaviors in young children. *Journal of Applied Behavior Analysis, 27,* 435–446.

Deacove, J. (1998). *Caves and claws.* Perth, ON, Canada: Family Pastimes.

Deacove, J. (1992). *Mountaineering.* Perth, ON, Canada: Family Pastimes.

Deacove, J. (1986). *Max (the cat).* Perth, ON, Canada: Family Pastimes.

Deacove, J. (1981). *Sleeping grump.* Perth, ON, Canada: Family Pastimes.

Deutsch, M. (1949). An experimental study of the effects of cooperation and competition on group process. *Human Relations, 2,* 199–231.

Garaigordobil, M., Maganio, C., & Etxeberria, J. (1996). Effects of a cooperative game program on socio-affective relations and group cooperative. *European Journal of Psychological Assessment, 12*(2), 141–152.

Knizia, R. (2000). *Lord of the rings.* Roseville, MN: Fantasy Flight Games.

Kolsbun, K., & Kolsbun, J. (1978). *Save the whales.* Santa Barbara, CA: Animal Town Game Company.

Mender, J., Kerr, R., & Orlick, T. (1982). A cooperative games program for learning disabled children. *International Journal of Sport Psychology, 13*(4), 222–233.

Orlick, T. (1981). Positive socialization via cooperative games. *Developmental Psychology, 17*(4), 426–429.

Tolkien, J. R. R. (1963). *The lord of the rings.* London: Allen & Unwin.

48

Chance Games

Introduction

A game of chance is an activity in which the outcome is determined by luck and not by skill. Games of chance have been a pastime and source of pleasure since ancient times and were commonly used to determine one's fate. For example, the Greeks and the Romans believed gods and goddesses had power over events and could interfere with the tossing of dice.

One of the earliest and most popular chance games played in ancient times was Knucklebones, a game similar to what we now call Jacks. The ankle or knucklebones of animals were used for this game. Players threw them into the air and caught as many as they could on the back of their hands or picked up as many bones as they could from the ground while one was in the air. In addition, knucklebones were often used for a gambling game similar to the game of dice. Because each side of a knucklebone is different, each side was given a value. The bones were thrown from a moderate height over the ground or a table and scores were determined. Romans often used knucklebones made from brass, silver, gold, ivory, marble, bronze, or glass to play this game, which they called Tali (Tali: Knuckle Bones, n.d.).

A well-known chance game for children, Snakes and Ladders (now called Chutes and Ladders) originated as a game based on morality called Vaikuntapaali or Paramapada Sopanam (the ladder to salvation). The game was called Leela and was invented by Hindu spiritual teachers to teach children about Karma and the effects of good versus bad deeds. The ladders represented virtues such as generosity, faith, and humility, and the snakes represented vices such as envy, anger, and stealing. The moral of the game was that good deeds result in salvation (Moksha) and evil deeds bring about rebirth in lower forms of life (Patamu). The number of

224

ladders on the game was less than the number of snakes as a reminder that the path of good is more difficult than the path of sin (Bell, 1983; Topsfield, 1985).

Rationale

Chance games offer a variety of benefits for children in play therapy that improve social, emotional, and cognitive functioning include:

- *Working alliance/relationship enhancement.* Because they are familiar to most children, chance games are an ideal way to engage children in treatment. They do not require the concentration needed for strategy games, which enables children and therapists to have spontaneous conversations and discussions of issues while playing them.

- *Diagnostic understanding.* Chance games are a valuable tool for assessing social–emotional functioning, self-esteem, social skills, and coping. While playing chance games with children, the therapist observes how the child interacts with the therapist (opponent), solves problems, and copes with frustration and disappointment. The therapist also notes the extent to which the child worries about winning, if cheating takes place, and whether he/she is able to enjoy the game.

- *Socialization/social skills.* Chance games require that the child follow directions, control impulses, take turns (reciprocity), and accept the frustration of losing. In addition, chance games often require face-to-face contact and verbal communication, which enhances comfort in social situations and improves communication skills.

- *Positive emotions.* Chance games are fun and provide an escape from stress and everyday problems. Playing games with an empathic therapist promotes a sense of hope and shows children that they can have fun even when problems arise. In addition, the realization that the therapist enjoys their company helps children internalize positive feelings about themselves, which fosters a sense of competence and well-being. Playing chance games with peers means that there is an equal likelihood that everyone will experience success, which fosters bonding with others.

- *Coping skills.* Since luck plays such a big role in chance games, they are an ideal tool for assessing and teaching coping skills related to winning, losing, and tolerating frustration associated with changes and mishaps that occur during the game. Chance games also provide a way for therapists to model and teach cooperation, compassion, good sportsmanship, and ways to deal with disappointing experiences.

- *Communication.* The fact that things change unexpectedly in chance games, despite one's effort, can serve as a metaphor for the fact that changes happen unexpectedly and by chance in real life. This makes chance games a great tool for discussing ways to cope with the losses and unexpected changes that happen in life.

Description

Ages

Four years and up. Chance games commonly include specific directions for playing. These can range in complexity depending on the game and the age for which the game is designed. Therapists may choose to adjust directions for the game to meet developmental needs of the children they work with.

Techniques

The following are our picks of the most classic, time-honored chance games for children.

Candy Land

First published by Hasbro in 1949, Candy Land is designed for children ages 3–6 years. The object of the game is to find King Kandy, the lost king of Candy Land, by traveling along a winding path of 134 spaces. Each space is colored red, green, blue, yellow, orange, or purple and five remaining spaces are named for places or characters. Players take turns removing the top card from a stack, showing one of six colors, and move their marker to the next space of that color. Some cards have two marks of a color, in which case the player moves his/her marker ahead to the second-next space of that color. The deck also has one card for each named location or character. Drawing these cards requires that the player move to that location on the board. This move can be forward or backward in this classic game. However, backward moves are ignored for younger players in the 2004 version of the game.

Sorry

This game by Hasbro for children ages 6 years and up is for two to four players. Each player starts the game with three pawns in the color that he/she chooses. Players take turns drawing cards to see how far they can move one of the candy-kiss-shaped pieces on the board. When players land on a slide, they can zip to the end and bump the opponents' pawns or their own. The game involves jumping over pawns, hiding in safety zones to get powers, and bumping back the opponents' pawns. The first person to get all three of their pawns from start to home is the winner.

War

Two or more players use a standard deck of 52 cards to play this game. It is suitable for children ages 6 years and up who are familiar with the ranking of playing cards from high to low (Ace, King, Queen, Jack, 10, 9, 8, etc.). Cards are equally distributed among players and are kept in a pile facedown. Players turn their top card faceup and put them on the table. The player with the highest-ranking card takes both cards and adds them to the bottom of his/her stack of cards. If the turned-up cards are equal, there is a war. The tied cards stay on the table and both players play the next card of their pile facedown and then another card faceup. Whoever has the higher of the new faceup cards wins the war and adds all six cards to the bottom of his/her stack. If the new faceup cards are equal as well, the war continues. The game continues until one player has all the cards and wins (McLeod, 2013).

Go Fish

A perennial favorite card game for two to four players, ages 4 years and up, it consists of 40 cards (10 sets of four matching fish). The dealer shuffles the cards and deals six to each player. The remaining cards are spread face down in the center of the table to create a pond. Starting with the player to the left of the dealer, each person takes a turn asking another player if he/she has a certain fish. If asked for a card he/she has, a player must hand over all of the cards of that fish. The asker then gets to take another turn. If a player has no cards of the requested fish, he/she responds, "Go fish." The asker then draws a card from the pile. If he/she draws the card he/she was requesting, the asker shows the card to the group as proof and takes another turn. Players try to form sets of four of a kind. When they do, the four cards are placed on the table face up. Play continues until all cards are matched. The player who makes the most sets wins.

Empirical Findings

This technique is in need of empirical research.

Applications

Chance games are an ideal technique for engaging children in treatment and are particularly helpful for shy, withdrawn, and slow-to-warm-up children who prefer familiar activities. In addition, chance games teach social skills such as cooperation, taking turns, and sportsmanship to children with behavior problems, developmental delays, and other social difficulties. They provide a way to help children who are overly competitive, have problems with impulse control, and have difficulties tolerating frustrations. In addition, the fun quality of chance games makes them a great tool for imparting joy and providing a break from reality for depressed and anxious children and those with histories of loss, abuse, or trauma.

References

Bell, R. C. (1983). *The boardgame book* (pp. 134–135). Reading, PA: Exeter Books.

McLeod, J. (2013, March 4). Card game rules war. Retrieved from *www.pagat.com*.

Tali: Knuckle Bones. (n.d.). Retrieved from *www.aerobiologicalengineering.com/wxk116/ Roman/BoardGames/tali.html*.

Topsfield, A. (1985). The Indian game of snakes and ladders. *Artibus Asiae*, 46(3), 203–226.

49

Squiggle Game

Introduction

One of the most famous play therapy techniques, created by British child psychiatrist Donald Winnicott (1971), is his squiggle game. A squiggle is any variation of a small line (wiggly, curved, wavy, or zigzagged).

Rationale

Winnicott found that not only did the squiggle game help build initial rapport with children who found the game to be fun (Berger, 1980), but it also furnished him with valuable information about the children's inner world, including internal conflicts. The squiggle game also provides therapists with opportunities to indirectly offer clients new ideas or solutions to their problems.

Description

Ages

Eight to 12 years.

Materials

White paper and pencils.

Techniques

Winnicott (1971) introduced the squiggle game to children by saying:

Let's play something. I know what I would like to play and I'll show you. This game that I like playing has no rules. I just take my pencil and go like that (he closes his eyes and draws a squiggle). You show me if that looks like anything to you or if you can make it into anything, and afterwards you do the same for me and I will see if I can make something of yours. (pp. 62–63)

Variations

Squiggle Drawing Game (Claman, 1980)

After completing a squiggle drawing, the child is asked to tell a story about it, and the therapist can ask questions about it. This procedure is repeated for the therapist. The therapist shares through his/her own drawings and stories his/her understanding of the child's problems and suggests possible solutions. The therapist's drawing should have a lesson or main idea that encourages the belief that the child can master his/her problems as well as suggesting a way to do so.

An adaptation of this is for the child's parent to draw a squiggle for the child to make a picture out of and tell a story about the picture. Then the child draws a squiggle and the parent follows the same procedure. Another variation is for the therapist and child to jointly select four of their squiggle pictures and collaborate in telling a story about them (i.e., take turns adding to the story line).

Empirical Findings

The squiggle game is in need of empirical research.

Applications

The squiggle game is designed to help establish rapport with school-age children early in therapy. It provides them with an opportunity to project unconscious material.

References

Berger, L. (1980). The Winnicott squiggle game: A vehicle for communicating with the school-aged child. *Pediatrics*, 66(60), 921–924.

Claman, L. (1980). The squiggle drawing game in child psychotherapy. *American Journal of Psychotherapy*, 34, 414–425.

Winnicott, D. W. (1971). *Therapeutic consultation in child psychiatry*. London: Hogarth Press.

Part Seven

OTHER TECHNIQUES

50

Desensitization Play

Introduction

Systematic desensitization is a well-known technique used by therapists to help children overcome fears and phobias. It is a type of counterconditioning approach developed by Joseph Wolpe (1958). The first step for a child presenting with a dog phobia, for instance, would be to establish a fear hierarchy by asking the child to rate the intensity of his/her fear to various levels of exposure to the feared object— for example, a puppy might result in a low fear rating by the child as compared with encountering a large dog. The next step is to identify an alternate response to a puppy that can counteract and lessen the child's fear, such as play. The third step is for the child, while playing, to be exposed to a small, friendly puppy so that the fun of playing overcomes the fear. Once this is successfully accomplished, the child would gradually be exposed to other dog situations on the fear hierarchy.

Rationale

Wolpe (1958) used the term *reciprocal inhibition* to refer to the phenomenon that certain psychological states are mutually exclusive. Thus, anxiety and joy cannot be experienced at the same time. So strong, positive affects experienced in play can serve to overcome anxiety and fear of the playing child. When two stimuli are systematically coupled, the presence of a stronger positive stimulus will change the child's experience of a fear-provoking negative stimulus. Accordingly, play and its positive qualities can be used as a means of systematic desensitization for a fearful child.

There are two main ways that play has been used to desensitize a child's fears and phobias. The first is the "emotive imagery" technique, a form of imaginal exposure. The second is the "emotive performances" technique, a form of real-life exposure to the feared object or situation.

Description

Ages

One year and up.

Techniques

Emotive Imagery

Emotive imagery is a form of visualization that was developed by Lazarus and Abramowitz (1962) and refers to imagery that produces strong positive feelings (e.g., happiness, power, courage) and other similar anxiety-inhibiting responses. It is typically part of a systematic desensitization procedure as the child engages in emotive imagery while anxiety-provoking items are gradually introduced. The more you feel positive affects in a fearful situation, the less afraid you feel because the positive affects counteract and weaken the negative affect (i.e., counterconditioning occurs). When counterconditioning occurs in fantasy it is called *in vitro exposure*; when it occurs in real life it is termed *in vivo exposure*.

Emotive imagery usually involves the therapist helping the child to develop a "story" about the child's favorite heroes helping him/her to be brave or fight back when the feared object (e.g., fear of the dark) is presented. The individually tailored story often focuses on imaginary special powers and using help from the super-hero to cope with the situation. Imagery incompatible with fear (super strength or powers, bravery) are triggered in the child by the story. Later, the child's parents prompt the child to use the individualized imagery scene to cope with real-life fearful situations. Alternately, images evoking feelings of happiness or mirth can be used through laughter-inducing images to countercondition fears—for example, Janet, age 6 years, presented with a strong fear of dogs. Her therapist used emotive imagery to help her see dogs as silly, slobbering animals rather than dangerous predators. This use of humor as a competing response is similar to the "party hat on monsters" technique (Crenshaw, 2001).

The emotive imagery technique has been particularly useful when the fear or phobia is imaginary and conventional *in vivo* exposure therapy is not possible (King, 1989). Researchers have found the emotive imagery technique to be generally effective for overcoming a client's fears (Shepard & Kuczynski, 2009).

Emotive Performances

Emotive performance is an example of an *in vivo* desensitization program. In this technique children ages 4–10 years engage in playful activities to engender positive emotions in order to counter fearful emotions, such as nighttime fears. Thus, to overcome a child's fear of the dark, therapists have had success training parents to play games with their child in his/her gradually darkened bedroom so that the positive emotions triggered by the play can serve to overcome the child's fear of a dark bedroom (Mendez & Garcia, 1996; Mikulas, Coffman, Dayton, & Maier, 1986; Santacruz, Mendez, & Sanchez-Meca, 2006).

Bentler (1962) presented a case study of a year-old girl who had slipped in the bathtub and subsequently exhibited an intense fear of water. To countercondition this fear, toys were placed in an empty bathtub and kitchen sink for her to play with. Water was gradually added to this play. Within a few months her fear of water was extinguished.

Empirical Findings

1. Fernandes and Arriaga (2010) investigated whether a clown intervention could reduce preoperative worries of children undergoing minor surgery. The results showed that when children were accompanied by their parents and a pair of clowns they were significantly less anxious than children who were just accompanied by their parents.

2. Fredrickson and Joiner (2002) reported that positive emotions such as mirth and joy enhance optimistic thinking, which leads to more creative problem solving. Research has also indicated that positive emotions have the ability to undo the effects of stress and encourage resiliency (Tugade & Fredrickson, 2004).

Applications

Desensitization play techniques are particularly effective with children who present with anxiety, phobias, night fears, or fears resulting from PTSD.

References

Bentler, P. M. (1962). An infant's phobia treated with reciprocal inhibition therapy. *Journal of Child Psychiatry and Psychology*, 3, 185–189.

Crenshaw, D. (2001). Party hats on monsters: Drawing strategies to enable children to master their fears. In H. G. Kaduson & C. E. Schaefer (Eds.), *101 more favorite play therapy techniques* (pp. 124–127). Lanham, MD: Rowman & Littlefield.

Fernandes, S., & Arriaga, P. (2010). The effects of clown intervention on worries and emotional responses in children undergoing surgery. *Journal of Health Psychology*, 15(3), 405–415.

Fredrickson, B., & Joiner, T. (2002). Positive emotions trigger upward spirals toward emotional well-being. *Psychological Science*, 13(2), 172–175.

King, N. (1989). Emotive imagery and children's night-time fears: A multiple baseline design evaluation. *Journal of Behavior Therapy and Experimental Psychiatry*, 20(2), 125–135.

Lazarus, A., & Abramovitz, A. (1962). The use of emotive imagery in the treatment of children's phobias. *Journal of Mental Science*, 198, 191–195.

Mendez, F., & Garcia, M. (1996). Emotive performances: A treatment package for children's phobias. *Child and Family Behavior Therapy*, 1(3), 19–34.

Mikulas, W., Coffman, M., Dayton, D., & Maier, P. (1986). Behavioral bibliotherapy and games for treating fear of the dark. *Child and Family Behavior Therapy, 7*(3), 1–8.

Santacruz, I., Mendez, F., & Sanchez-Meca, J. (2006). Play therapy applied by parents for children with darkness phobia: Comparison of two programs. *Child and Family Behavior Therapy, 1,* 19–35.

Shepherd, L., & Kuczynski, A. (2009). The use of emotive imagery and behavioral techniques for a 10-year-old boy's nocturnal fear of ghosts and zombies. *Clinical Case Studies, 8,* 99–11.

Tugade, M., & Fredrickson, B. (2004). Resilient individuals use positive emotions to bounce back from negative emotional experiences. *Personality and Social Psychology, 88*(2), 320–333.

Wolpe, J. (1958). *Psychotherapy by reciprocal inhibition.* Stanford, CA: Stanford University Press.

51

Laughter Play

Introduction

Laughter is an important and beneficial aspect of play because it promotes joy and a sense of well-being. Unfortunately, most people do not get enough laughter in their lives, especially clients suffering from various forms of psychopathology. Albert Ellis (1977) was one of the first therapists to advocate the use of laughter and humor in psychotherapy. He often used humorous comments to challenge a client's irrational beliefs. Laughter therapy has become a growing movement that seeks to help clients of all ages benefit from the many healing powers of mirthful laughter (Provine, 2001).

Rationale

Research findings on the psychological benefits of laughter can be summarized as follows:

> Laughter (1) reduces stress, anxiety, tension, and counter-acts depression symptoms; (2) elevates mood, self-esteem, hope, energy, and vigor; (3) enhances memory, creative thinking, and problem-solving; (4) improves interpersonal interaction, relationships, attraction, and closeness; (5) increases friendliness, helpfulness, and builds group identity, solidarity, and cohesiveness; (6) promotes psychological well-being; (7) improves quality of life and patient care; and (8) intensifies mirth and is contagious. (Mora-Ripoll, 2011, p. 172)

Among the therapeutic powers of laughter are:

- Cathartic release of anger, anxiety, and boredom (Provine, 2001).
- Increase in feelings of happiness (Neuhoff & Schaefer, 2002).
- Enhanced connection to others and fosters group cohesion (Ayers, Beyea, Godfrey, & Harper, 2005).

- Reduction of interpersonal conflict.
- Strengthening of resiliency.

Description

Ages

Four years and up.

Technique

Make Me Laugh

VanFleet (2001) describes the make-me-laugh technique as follows. The therapist states that the players (the therapist and the child in individual therapy; or the child and another child in group therapy) will take turns trying to make the other laugh or smile. The straight-faced player starts the game by gruffly saying, "Make me laugh." He/she must keep a serious face, maintain eye contact for the duration of turn, and under no circumstances laugh or smile.

The other player must then do whatever he/she can to try and get the straight-faced person to smile or laugh. This player may not physically touch the other but can move close to make faces, tell jokes, utter strange noises, or engage in any silly antics that might trigger laughter (e.g., contorted facial expressions, or clucking and flapping like a chicken).

The make-me-laugh technique can be used for brief periods over several sessions. A child's participation in this game must be voluntary and never forced. Make me laugh is a useful technique for children who, for whatever reason, rarely laugh or smile. Typically, children laugh about 400 times a day.

Variations

Hospital Clowning

This is a program in health care facilities involving visits from specially trained clowns. The hospital visits of these "clown doctors" have been shown to help in lifting children's moods with a joyful atmosphere of smiles, laughter, and fun. They help children adapt to their surroundings and distract them from frightening medical procedures.

Laughter Yoga

Since the body cannot distinguish between genuine and simulated laughter, Madan Kataria (2005) of Bombay, India, created Laughter Yoga clubs so adults across the world could enjoys the benefits of laughter. The laughter yoga technique includes four elements: clapping in rhythm to "Ho-ho-ha-ha-ha"; breathing; stretching, and child-like play and laughter exercises. A typical laughter yoga session entails about 20 minutes of laughter.

Parent–Child Tickling Game

Tickling games are interpersonal activities involving tickling one person by another (e.g., tickling the bottom of another person's feet with a feather). You cannot tickle yourself so you need the help of someone you trust. Tickling is probably the most ancient and effective way to evoke laughter in someone and thus increase his/her positive affect and connection to you. The object of parent–child tickling is to generate mirthful laughter in the child that facilitates bonding. The most ticklish areas of our bodies are, in descending order: underarms, waist, ribs, feet, knees, throat, neck, and palms.

Empirical Findings

1. Panksepp (2007) found that the positive state of mind that results from laughing makes us more likely to engage in friendly interactions with others.

2. Neuhoff and Schaefer (2002) reported that just 1 minute of simulated laughter increased feelings of happiness in college students.

3. Nevo and Shapira (1989) found that pediatric dentists routinely use a variety of playful, humorous techniques to alleviate anxiety of children in their dental setting.

4. Vagnoli (2005) reported that visits from clown doctors who played magic tricks, games, and performed puppet shows 30 minutes before a procedure reduced the preoperative anxiety of hospitalized children.

5. Golan, Tighe, Dobija, Perel, and Keidan (2009) found that medically trained clowns significantly alleviated preoperative anxiety in children ages 3–8 years undergoing outpatient surgery.

Applications

Clients experiencing stress, anxiety, tension, depression, attachment issues, and poor social relationships are particularly appropriate candidates for laughter therapy, either individually or in groups.

References

Ayers, L., Beyea, S., Godfrey, M., & Harper, D. (2005). Quality improvement learning collaboratives. *Quality Management in Health Care, 14*, 234–247.
Ellis, A. (1977). Fun as psychotherapy. *Rational Living, 2*(1), 2–6.

Golan, G., Tighe, P., Dobija, N., Perel, A., & Keidan, I. (2009). Clowns for the prevention of preoperative anxiety in children: A randomized controlled trial. *Pediatric Anesthesia, 19,* 262–266.

Kataria, M. (2005). Laughter Clubs. Available at *www.laughteryoga.org.*

Mora-Ripoli, R. (2011). Potential health benefits of simulated laughter: A narrative review of the literature and recommendations for future research. *Complementary Therapies, 19*(3), 170–177.

Neuhoff, C., & Schaefer, C. E. (2002). Effects of laughter, smiling and howling on mood. *Psychological Reports, 91,* 1079–1080.

Nevo, O., & Shapira, J. (1989). The use of humor by pediatric dentists. *Journal of Children in Contemporary Society, 20*(1–2), 171–178.

Panksepp, J. (2007). Neuroevolutionary sources of laughter and social play: Modeling primal human laughter in laboratory rats. *Behavioural Brain Research, 182*(2), 231–244.

Provine, R. (2001). *Laughter: A scientific investigation.* New York: Penguin Books.

Vagnoli, L. (2005). Clown doctors as a treatment for preoperative anxiety in children: A randomized, prospective study. *Journal of the American Academy of Pediatrics,* e563–e567.

VanFleet, R. (2001). Make me laugh. In H. G. Kaduson & C. E. Schaefer (Eds.), *101 more favorite play therapy techniques* (pp. 203–206). Northvale, NJ: Jason Aronson.

52

Stress Inoculation Play

Introduction

Stress inoculation therapy is an approach developed by psychologist Donald Meichenbaum (1985) to help people develop resiliency against the effects of stress through a procedure involving preexposure to stressful situations. The use of the term *inoculation* is based on the idea that a psychotherapist is inoculating or preparing a client to become resistant to the effects of upcoming stressors in a manner similar to how a vaccination works to make patients resistant to the effects of a particular disease. The procedure provides child clients the opportunity to practice in play coping skills until they become overlearned and easy to use.

Rationale

Rather than shielding a child from knowledge and worry about upcoming stressful experiences, such as starting school, or a medical procedure, a more adaptive approach is to prepare the child by providing information about it. This is Janis's (1958) theory of stress inoculation and the "work of worrying." The work of worrying is defined as a coping strategy in which inner preparation through worry increases the tolerance for subsequent threats (Burstein & Meichenbaum, 1979). Providing a child with details about what to expect during a stressful event makes the strange familiar and thus reduces the fear of the unknown. It also gives the child time to generate and practice ways to cope with the stressful experience. The moderate amount of anxiety triggered by the preparatory work of worrying should prevent severe emotional distress during the actual event.

241

Description

Ages

Four years and up.

Techniques

The anticipatory anxiety aroused in a child by any future, known, stressful event can be reduced by having the child play out the event in advance. Thus, a miniature, school play set (teacher, students, school bus, classroom, etc.) can be used by the therapist to model such activities as the ride to school, greeting the teacher, hanging up coats, and so on. By demonstrating with miniature toys exactly what to expect, the play therapist can make the strange school situation more familiar and thus less scary. In addition to providing information and support, the therapist can teach coping skills for handling the situation. A similar approach is to provide a child facing surgery with details of the procedure and medical toys/outfits to play it out a few days in advance.

Empirical Findings

1. Hodgins and Lander (1997) found that 27% of children lacking formal preparation who were undergoing venipuncture reported anxiety due to the unknown aspects of the procedure.

2. Numerous studies have shown the stress inoculation play technique to be particularly effective in reducing the anxiety of children prior to surgery (Athanassiadou, Giannakopoulos, Kolaitis, Tsiantis, & Christogiorgos, 2012; Li, Lopez, & Lee, 2007; Lockwood, 1970) and hospitalization (Jolly, 1976).

Applications

The stress inoculation play technique can be used prior to any future event that may cause anxiety for the child, including:

- A child who will be hospitalized.
- A child who will be starting school/camp.
- A child who will be moving to a new home.
- A child who will be going to the barber for his first haircut.
- A child who will be going to the doctor/dentist.
- A child about to meet a new sibling.

References

Athanassiadou, E., Giannakopoulos, G., Kolaitis, G., Tsiantis, J., & Christogiorgos, S. (2012). Preparing the child facing surgery: The use of play therapy. *Psychoanalytic Social Work*, *19*, 91–100.

Burstein, S., & Meichenbaum, D. (1979). The work of worrying in children undergoing surgery. *Journal of Abnormal Child Psychology*, *7*(2), 121–132.

Hodgins, M., & Lander, J. (1997). Children's coping with venipuncture. *Journal of Pain and Symptom Management*, *13*, 274–285.

Janis, I. L. (1958). *Psychological stress*. New York: Wiley.

Jolly, J. D. (1976). Preparing children for hospital. *Nursing Times*, *72*, 1532–1533.

Li, H., Lopez, V., & Lee, T. (2007). Effects of preoperative therapeutic play on outcomes of school-age children undergoing day surgery. *Research in Nursing and Health*, *30*, 320–332.

Lockwood, N. L. (1970). The effect of situational doll play upon the preoperative stress reactions of hospitalized children. *American Nursing Association Bulletin*, *9*, 113–120.

Meichenbaum, D. (1985). *Stress inoculation training*. Elmsford, NY: Pergamon Press.

53

Reenactment Play

Introduction

Sigmund Freud (1922) was the first person to notice that through the use of play children can relive stressful or traumatic events in a safe environment and gain a sense of power and control over them. Through repetitive play reexperiences, a child can gradually mentally digest, abreact/release negative feelings, and develop a sense of mastery over disturbing thoughts and feelings (Waelder, 1932). Piaget (1962) also proposed that make-believe play provides children with opportunities to reproduce in fantasy real-life problems, to work out adaptive solutions, and thus ameliorate negative emotions.

David Levy (1939) was one of the first child clinicians to introduce a form of structured play therapy, which he called "release therapy." The goal of release therapy is to help children express their thoughts and feeling after experiencing a specific stressful or traumatic event. Although children are free to choose how they want to play, the play materials are limited and preselected by the therapist to encourage children to play out their traumatic experiences. Levy structured play sessions by providing hospital-related dolls and toys for a child dealing with the stress of being in a hospital. He would then ask the child to talk about or show what is happening to the boy doll in the hospital bed.

Rationale

It is common for children to experience stressful or traumatic events, which result in feelings of confusion, helplessness, vulnerability, and fear. Parents may not know how to help children with these emotions and may believe that it is better not to talk about traumatic events. Rather than encouraging a child to bury and forget about a trauma memory that will likely continue to intrude into consciousness, it is healthier to help the child reenact the stressful event in play where he/she can repeat and slowly mentally digest it, express negative affect, and create a satisfactory ending, and thus gain a sense of mastery over it.

Underlying reenactment play is Sigmund Freud's (1922) theory of repetition compulsion. The idea is that given relevant play materials and a safe environment, the child will replay a stressful/traumatic event repeatedly until he/she is able to mentally assimilate the distressing thoughts and feelings. The repetition also allows abreaction to occur—that is, full expression of emotional reactions to the traumatic experience (Terr, 2003).

Description

Ages

Four to 12 years.

Techniques

Children have a natural tendency to cope with traumas through play—for example, many children were observed building towers with blocks after viewing TV images of the horror of 9/11 and then crashing toy airplanes into the towers. In another instance (Goldman, 1995), children who experienced a gunman—Patrick Purdy—shooting other children on their school playground before killing himself subsequently were observed playing a game they created called "Purdy." This game involved running in different directions on the school playground in a reenactment of the actual event. Other versions involved their playing with guns and killing Purdy. Such reenactment play, also called abreaction play, is one of the most potent ways children cope with the experience of specific traumas and stressors (Prendiville, 2014; Terr, 1990).

In a reenactment play therapy session with a child who recently experienced a car accident in which a parent was seriously injured, the therapist would prearrange the playroom so that the only play objects available for the child to play with are ones related to the accident (e.g., toy cars, traffic signs, ambulances, police cars, medical equipment, doctors, and police). The child would then engage in free play to develop a sense of control over the accident that he did not have in real life. Typically, the child will need to repeat this reenactment play in subsequent sessions to fully assimilate and master the stressful experience.

Empirical Findings

1. Six months after a major earthquake devastated six villages in Italy, Galante and Foa (1986) conducted pay therapy with children from one of the two hardest-hit villages. During seven monthly group sessions, children in grades one through four were given the opportunity to reenact the earthquake experience in their play and express their feelings about it. To re-create the quake they shook tables to topple miniature toy houses. They then pretended to be firefighters or rescue workers who helped the survivors and rebuilt the village. Compared with children in the untreated village, anxiety symptoms were significantly reduced in the children who received reenactment play. Treatment gains were maintained at an 18-month follow-up.

2. Saylor, Swenson, and Powell (1992) reported that preschoolers, after Hurricane Hugo, tended on their own initiative to repeatedly play out themes related to the hurricane. For example, 8 weeks after the storm, a mother reported that her 4-year-old son repeatedly replayed the Hugo storm with every medium available, including broccoli spears at the dinner table, which represented the trees being ravaged again and again by the winds that reached 175 miles per hour.

Applications

This technique is designed for use with children who have experienced a single-incident stressful or traumatic experience, such as a car accident, dog bite, medical procedure, or abuse. It has been conducted with child clients in individual, family, and group therapy.

Contraindications

This release therapy technique is not appropriate for children who have or are experiencing multiple traumas or reoccurring traumas, such as ongoing sexual abuse.

References

Freud, S. (1922). *Beyond the pleasure principle*. London: International Psychoanalytical Press.
Galante, R., & Foa, E. (1986). An epidemiological study of psychic trauma and treatment effectiveness of children after a natural disaster. *Journal of the American Academy of Child Psychiatry, 25,* 357–363.
Goldman, D. (1995). *Intelligence: Why it can matter more than IQ*. New York: Bantam Books.
Levy, D. (1922). Trends in therapy: The evolution and present status of treatment approaches to behavior and personality problems: III. Release therapy. *American Journal of Orthopsychiatry, 9*(1), 713–736.
Piaget, J. (1962). *Play, dreams, and imitation*. New York: Norton.
Prendiville, E. (2014). Abreaction. In C. E. Schaefer & A. A. Drewes (Eds.), *The therapeutic powers of play: 20 core agents of change* (pp. 83–102). Hoboken, NJ: Wiley.

Saylor, C., Swenson, C., & Powell, P. (1992). Hurricane Hugo blows down the broccoli: Pre-schoolers' post-disaster play and adjustment. *Child Psychiatry and Human Development*, 22(3), 139–149.

Terr, L. (1990). *Too scared to cry: Psychic trauma in childhood*. New York: Basic Books.

Terr, L. (2003). "Wild child": How three principles of healing organized 12 years of psycho-therapy. *Journal of the American Academy of Child and Adolescent Psychiatry*, 42(12), 401–409.

Waelder, R. (1932). The psychoanalytic theory of play. *Psychoanalytic Quarterly*, 2, 208–224.

54

Hide-and-Seek Play

> Just as mommy disappears and reappears in the game of peekaboo, mommy now can literally disappear, but the toddler knows she still exists and will return. She can create mommy's image in her mind's eye. . . .
>
> —THE SUCCESSFUL PARENT WEBSITE

Introduction

Hide-and-Seek is a children's game that has been played for many generations. In the traditional game, one player, the seeker, covers his/her eyes and counts while one or more players hide. After counting to a certain number, the seeker attempts to find the hider(s). Children in play therapy often introduce hide-and-seek games spontaneously during their sessions. They may hide and wait for the therapist to find them; ask the therapist to hide so they can show their skill at seeking; create treasure hunt scenarios in the sandtray; hide objects in the playroom or sandtray; or hide behind sunglasses, masks, or costumes. Similarly, children may introduce peekaboo games by pretending to disappear and popping out from behind an object to surprise the therapist.

Themes of disappearance and reappearance are central in Hide-and-Seek and Peekaboo, and are frequently played by children with attachment issues and histories of loss, separation, and trauma. These games often convey a need to be in control, anxiety about aloneness, avoidance of intimacy, ambivalent attachment styles, and difficulties with internalizing the pleasure of reunions (Allan & Pare, 1997).

Rationale

Hide-and-Seek has many therapeutic benefits, including:

248

- *Object permanence*. Infant research highlights that early experiences with disappearance and reappearance influence object permanence, an understanding that objects, events, and people continue to exist even when they not are seen, heard, or touched (Piaget, 1954). In addition, separations and reunions play a crucial role on object constancy; the child's understanding that he/she is separate from the caregiver and that put of sight is not out of mind. According to Mahler, Pine, and Bergman (1975), children who achieve object constancy have an internalized representation of the caregiver who provides them with support, comfort, and self-confidence. Children who lack object constancy tend to struggle with insecurity and low self-esteem. Separation/reunion games such as Hide-and-Seek and Peekaboo are a great way to help children practice coping with separation from their mothers (Israelievitch, 2008).

- Disappearance and reappearance games begin in infancy with the game Peekaboo. Research has shown that this game, played by infants around the world, helps children attain object permanence (Fernald & O'Neill, 1993; Lacy, 2014). Playing Peekaboo and Hide-and-Seek with a responsive therapist gives children an opportunity to play out needs to separate and reunite and helps them internalize a sense of safety/comfort in their separateness. This enables children to make the shift from needing the physical presence of adults to building an internal sense of security (Allan & Pare, 1997; Israelievitch, 2008).

- Ainsworth, Blehar, Waters, and Wall (1978) noted that securely attached children know that their needs will be met when they seek comfort and closeness from attachment figures. These children have a secure base from which to explore their world. In contrast, insecurely attached children lack this sense of comfort, confidence, and security. Hide-and-seek play is a natural way for children to develop secure attachments. This game helps children see that other people are trustworthy and reliable, that they will not be forgotten, and that they are worthy of being found. Disappearance and reappearance games also reassure children that people in relationships can separate but they will later come together.

- *Attachment*. Both Hide-and-Seek and Peekaboo are enjoyable games. They provide laughter and joy, which enhance attachments. Caspar Addyman, director of the Baby Laughter Project in London, has found that Peekaboo is the funniest game for babies (Philby, 2012).

- *Self-expression*. By playing Hide-and-Seek, a child may be able to express what is unspeakable and unconscious because of early attachment failure.

- *Therapeutic relationship*. Vollmer (2009) argued that Hide-and-Seek satisfies children's need for autonomy and conveys a message that they are free to explore and venture away. In addition, children benefit from being pursued because it shows that they are cared for. Allan and Pare (1997) wrote:

> We have noticed that there is a range of feelings embedded in the drama of the game: there is the arousal of the child's body, the thrill of being wanted and sought, the

pleasure of surprise, the power of controlling the interaction, the anxiety of loss, the pain over the loss of the loved one, the delight and relief of reunion, the fear of aloneness, the conquering of that fear, the great pleasure of confusing an adult and ultimately the empowerment that comes with magic. (p. 160)

Description

Ages

Infancy and up.

Techniques

Behavioral Hide-and-Seek

Allan and Pare (1997) note that it is important to create spaces within the play-room that facilitate playing the game. This might include angling a sofa away from the wall, using full-length drapes, or creating a cubby with curtains and blankets in a corner of the playroom. In addition, it is important that the therapist remain observant to Hide-and-Seek themes during children's play, which may be verbal or nonverbal—for instance, children may hide under a desk or say, "Pretend you can't see me." When these invitations occur, it is important that the therapist convey emotional reactions that show dismay and disappointment that the child is miss-ing, apprehension that he/she won't be found, sadness because he/she is missed, and delight when they are reunited (Allan & Pare, 1997).

Imaginary Hide-and-Seek (Prat, 2001)

The child thinks of an imaginary place to hide in the therapist's office or play-room—for example, "On top of the bookcase," "Under the cushions," "In the dollhouse," and "In the turtle puppet." Once the child has selected a hiding place, he/she says "Ready," and responds with "Hot" and "Cold" to the therapist's guesses. The therapist then takes a turn selecting a mental hiding place for the child to guess.

Feelings Hide-and-Seek

This therapeutic version of Hide-and-Seek (Kenney-Noziska, 2008) is a technique that facilitates emotional expression. To prepare for the activity, the therapist writes feelings on index cards and hides them around the playroom. When the child finds the cards, he/she discusses the feeling and a time it was experienced.

Peekaboo Play

Flap books as well as toddler toys such as Jack-in-the-Box, Peek-a-Boo Panda by Melissa and Doug, and computer apps such as Peekaboo Friends by Night and

Day Studios, Inc., promote peekaboo play and thus strengthen a sense of object permanence in infants and young children.

Sardines

This group game is similar to Hide-and-Seek except that one child hides and everyone else seeks. When you find the hiding person you hide with him/her until everyone is hiding together.

Empirical Findings

This technique is in need of empirical research.

Applications

Hide-and-seek and peekaboo games are especially therapeutic for children with insecure attachments due to trauma, abandonment, adoption, death, or divorce. Many of these children feel unimportant, unwanted, and unworthy of being found. They are drawn to Hide-and-Seek because it enables them to externalize these feelings and master the wounds associated with them. Doing so with an emotionally attuned therapist provides new experiences that help these children internalize a sense of being important and valued. This increases confidence, security, and self-esteem. Even so-called securely attached children may express a need for comfort and reassurance during periods of parental separation by playing separation/reunion games.

References

Ainsworth, M. D. S., Blehar, M. C., Waters, E., & Wall, S. (1978). *Patterns of attachment: A psychological study of the strange situation*. Hillsdale, NJ: Erlbaum.
Allan, J., & Pare, M. A. (1997). Hide-and-seek in play therapy. In H. G. Kaduson & C. E. Schaefer (Eds.), *101 play therapy techniques* (pp. 158–162). Northvale, NJ: Jason Aronson.
Fernald, A., & O'Neill, D. K. (1993). Peek-a-boo across cultures: How mothers and infants play with voices, faces, and expectations. In K. B. MacDonald (Ed.), *Parent–child play: Descriptions and implications*. Albany: State University of New York Press.
Israelievitch, G. (2008). Hiding and seeking and being found: Reflections on the hide-and-seek game in the clinical playroom. *Journal of Infant, Child, and Adolescent Psychotherapy*, 7, 58–76.
Kenney-Noziska, S. (2008). *Techniques–techniques–techniques: Play-based activities for children, adolescents, and families*. West Conshokocken, PA: Infinity.
Lacy, A. (2014, March 11). Peek-a-boo: A window on baby's brain. Retrieved from *www.bbc.com/news/health-24553877*.
Mahler, M. S., Pine, F., & Bergman, A. (1975). *The psychological birth of the human infant*. New York: Basic Books.

Philby, C. (2012). Peekaboo!: Why do babies laugh? Retrieved from *www.iol.co.za/lifestyle/family/baby-toddler/peekaboo-why-do-babies-laugh-1.1420745#.VNF9Lyx0xjo*.

Piaget, J. (1954). *The origins of intelligence*. New York: Basic Books.

Prat, R. (2001), Imaginary hide and seek: A technique for opening up a psychic space in child psychotherapy. *Journal of Child Psychotherapy, 27*(2), 175–196.

Vollmer, S. (2009, December 23). Hide and seek. *Psychology Today*. Retrieved from *www.psychologytoday.com/blog/learning-play/200912/hide-and-seek*.

55

Magic Tricks

All magic is about transformation . . . the performance magician is
telling you that you are the magician in your own life. You are the
agent of transformation, your own transformation.
—EUGENE BURGER

Introduction

The art of illusion has fascinated people throughout the world since ancient times.
Magicians performed for Pharaohs as far back as 5000 B.C.E. Primitive drawings
of sorcerers can be found on cave walls in Europe. Magicians performed in the
streets of ancient Greece and Rome. In 1584, Jean Prévost published the first book
on practical magic, *La Première Partie des Subtiles et Plaisantes Inventions* [*The
First Part of Subtle and Pleasant Tricks*]. At that time, street magicians flourished
all over the world, from English fairgrounds to tiny villages in India.

Jean Eugene Robert-Houdini, also known as the "Father of Modern Magic,"
brought magic from the street and circus shows to elegant Parisian stages and
drawing rooms in the mid-1800s. Around the same time, John Henry Anderson
pioneered the art of magic in London. In the early 1900s prestigious organizations
such as the Society of American Magicians in New York City and The Magic
Circle in London were formed to promote the art of stage magic. Since that time,
magic shows have been performed on stages and television shows throughout the
world. They are a common source of entertainment at children's parties and social
gatherings (All About Magicians.com, n.d.).

In 1988, award-winning illusionist Kevin Spencer suffered a head and spinal
cord injury and spent several months in physical and occupational therapy. When
he regained functioning, he and his wife developed the foundation of the Healing of Magic, a program to help patients regain physical skills while increasing
motivational levels and self-esteem. In 1977, Howard published the first book on
the use of magic in psychotherapy with children. Today, "magic therapy" is used

in hospitals, rehabilitation facilities, and schools in many countries (Healing of Magic, 2014).

Rationale

Children are inherently interested in magic tricks because they are mysterious, alluring, and challenging. This makes them an ideal tool for play therapy. Magic tricks have several therapeutic benefits:

• *Rapport building.* Since magic is an intriguing activity, it is an excellent resource for engaging resistant children in treatment and for establishing a therapeutic alliance (Bow, 1988; Frey, 2008). In addition, magic tricks are nonthreatening and fun. They show the child that therapy can be an enjoyable experience that can enhance motivation to continue in therapy (Stehouwer, 1983).

• *Metaphorical teaching.* Magic tricks can be used as a metaphor or symbol to convey messages about issues such as the power of change, transforming negative into positive, the importance of looking beyond the obvious, and the virtue of patience (Bow, 1988). Magic tricks help children understand that when things seem impossible, additional knowledge can make them work out. Although the child may feel helpless, the therapist can help him/her find new ways to cope and resolve issues.

• *Competence.* Teaching the child the "secret" of the trick is empowering, boosts the child's self-esteem, and instills confidence that the child can solve other life problems.

• *Instillation of hope.* Magic tricks can symbolize optimism, the possibility of change, and suggest that solutions to problems are not always as complicated as they appear.

• *Group cohesion.* They are an effective ice-breaker for new groups.

• *Executive functioning.* Magic tricks require concentration, planning, memory, perception, eye–hand coordination, motor planning, sequencing, and the ability to follow simple and complex directions.

• *Positive emotions.* Magic tricks are interesting, challenging, and fun. They tend to elevate one's mood.

Description

Ages

Four years and up.

Techniques

Gilroy (2001) provided a list of factors to consider when choosing magic tricks for play therapy. He noted that they should be simple, easy to learn and use, examinable, have few pieces, and appropriate for repeated use. In addition, they should be made for close-up magic, offer quick, easy setup, capture the interest of children, and promote interaction. See Stehouwer (1983) for a description of several very simple magic tricks that can be easily mastered by therapists and children.

General guidelines for using magic tricks in play therapy have been previously published (Frey, 2008; Gilroy, 2001; Pogue, 1998) and include:

• *Consent.* To prevent children from feeling manipulated or tricked, always obtain children's consent before doing a magic trick. Thus, you might ask if the child would like to see you do some magic.

• *Sharing.* When children ask, show the secret of the trick after performing it. This helps to build trust and fosters a therapeutic alliance. Doing so is especially important when working with suspicious or guarded children. Children below the age of 6 years are usually interested in a magic trick for the sake of the delight they experience from seeing the trick. However, children ages 6 years and up tend to be very interested in how the trick was done (Stehouwer, 1983).

• *Age appropriateness.* It is important to use magic tricks that are age appropriate and that the child can touch, examine, and master.

• *Social interaction.* Magic tricks should facilitate interaction between the therapist and child. Involving the child in the magic trick fosters this process. Always avoid "trickiness," such as fake cards.

• *Metaphorical communication.* Magic tricks can be used as embedded metaphors that convey messages to further the child's treatment and personal growth, such as things often seem impossible until someone shows you an alternate way to accomplish them.

• *Safe and accessible.* Use tricks that are done with simple, accessible materials that the child can easily obtain. Do not use dangerous materials. In addition, it is important not to use magic with children who have poor reality testing or psychosis.

Specific Magic Tricks

• *D'lite.* Gilroy (2001) introduced this trick for group counseling with children ages 5 years and up. This trick is available in most magic stores and can be used to teach tolerance, respect, conflict resolution and the uselessness of putdowns. The therapist presents two lights to the child, one in each hand. He/she raises his/her right-hand light and says, "This is your candle." The therapist raises his/her left-hand light and says, "This is my candle." Both lights are then held close together and the therapist says, "As you can see, your candle and mine are glowing at the same brightness, don't you agree?" The group is instructed to focus on the left candle (his/her candle) and the therapist blows out the candle on the right. The therapist says, "I've just blown out your candle and you didn't see my candle glow any brighter, did you?" The right candle is then relit and the group is instructed to focus on it. The therapist blows out the candle in the left hand and says, "My candle has just been blown out; yours didn't glow any brighter either, did it?"

• Frey (2008) introduced the following three magic tricks for young children ages 5 years and up to establish a therapeutic alliance, increase insight regarding the possibility of change, and enhance creative problem solving.

1. *Jumping Rubber Band Trick.* The therapist tells the child that he/she will make a rubber band jump from his/her small finger to the fore or middle finger. The therapist then puts the band on his/her small finger, folds all four fingertips under the inside of the band and then folds the fingers toward the palm. The band leaps from the small fingers to the fore and middle fingers.

2. *Drink-the-Water Trick.* The therapist places a glass of water in his/her outstretched right hand and asks the child to hold his/her right arm with both hands. The child is told that despite his/her effort to hold down the therapist's arm, the therapist can lift the glass and drink the water. When the child tightens his/her grip, the therapist reaches out with his/her left arm, lifts the glass, and drinks the water.

3. *Straw-in-the-Potato Trick.* The therapist asks the child to push a straw into a potato. When the child cannot do so, the therapist tries. The therapist then folds over one end of the straw, grips it in his/her hand, takes the other end of the straw, and pushes it into the potato. The straw now penetrates the potato because the air was compressed when the end of the straw was folded.

Variation

Therapeutic Metaphor

A magic trick can be used as a metaphor for life experiences, such as when you feel something is impossible to accomplish but, with guidance, you discover it is not; or when you feel you have free choice when in reality the deck is stacked against you.

Empirical Findings

1. Vagnoli, Caprilli, Robiglio, and Mestri (2005) compared presurgery anxiety levels in 40 children ages 5–12 years who were about to have minor surgery. Half of the children had a clown who performed magic tricks and parent along

while waiting for surgery and during the delivery of anesthesia. The other half had only a parent and medical staff present. The results shows that the children who had a clown or magician present until they fell asleep experienced significantly less presurgery anxiety and, consequently, required less anesthesia.

2. Peretz and Gluck (2005) examined the use of magic to improve cooperation in children who refused to enter the dentist office and sit in the dental chair. Seventy children, ages 3–6 years were randomly assigned to the test or control group. Children in the test group were shown a magic trick using a magic book (pictures erased magically and then drawn again) prior to being encouraged to sit in the chair. Children in the control group were told to sit in the chair and were provided positive reinforcement for doing so. The researchers examined the amount of time it took children to sit in the dental chair; their level of cooperation with X-rays, and their rating on the Frankl's behavior category. The amount of time spent to get children to sit in the dental chair was significantly shorter in the magic group and X-rays were taken in significantly more children than in the control. The magic group were also more cooperative, as measured by the Frankl.

Applications

Magic tricks are an ideal way to establish rapport and increase motivation for therapy in children and adolescents, particular those who are resistant to engaging in treatment. They are an excellent tool for teaching attention skills to children with ADHD, oppositional defiant disorder, difficulties with impulsivity, and limited frustration tolerance. Finally, magic tricks are useful tools in group counseling where they can help foster group cohesion.

Contraindications

Magic tricks can be used with almost all children except those children who are paranoid or psychotic, where magic may blur the distinction between fantasy and reality.

References

All About Magicians.com. (n.d.). History of magicians—timeline. Retrieved from *www.all-about-magicians.com/history-of-magicians.html*.

Bow, J. N. (1988). Treating resistant children. *Child and Adolescent Social Work*, 5(1), 3–15.

Frey, D. (2008). Therapeutic magic tricks. In L. Lowenstein (Ed.), *Assessment and treatment activities for children, adolescents, and families* (Vol. 1, pp. 34–35). Ontario, Canada: Champion Books.

Gilroy, B. D. (2001). Using magic therapeutically with children. In H. G. Kaduson & C. E.

Schaefer (Eds.), *101 more favorite play therapy techniques* (pp. 429–438). Northvale, NJ: Jason Aronson.

Healing of Magic. (2014). What is the healing of magic? Retrieved from *www.magictherapy. com*.

Howard, T. (1977). *How to use magic in psychotherapy with children*. Long Beach, MS: Emerald.

Peretz, B., & Gluck, G. (2005). Magic trick: A behavioural strategy for the management of strong willed children. *International Journal of Pediatric Dentistry, 15*, 429–436.

Pogue, D. (1998). *Magic for dummies*. New York: Hungry Minds.

Stehouwer, R. C. (1983). Using magic to establish rapport and improve motivation in psychotherapy with children: Theory, issues, and technique. *Psychotherapy in Private Practice, 1*(2), 85–94.

Vagnoli, L., Caprilli, S., Robiglio, B. A., & Mestri, A. (2005). Clown doctors as a treatment for preoperative anxiety in children: A randomized, prospective study. *Pediatrics, 116*(4), 563–567.

56

Feeling Faces

> Unexpressed emotions will never die. They are buried alive and will
> come forth later in uglier ways.
>
> —SIGMUND FREUD

Introduction

Harvey Ball, an American graphic artist, created the first yellow smiley face in
1963. Ball was commissioned by the State Mutual Life Assurance Company (now
called Allmerica Financial Corporation) to create a design to be used on posters,
buttons, and signs to raise employee morale. The smiley face gained huge popularity in the years that followed. In the early 1970s, Bernard and Murray Spain, own-
ers of two Philadelphia card shops, added the slogan "Have a Happy Day" to the
smile, copyrighted the revised mark, and produced a wide variety of novelty items.
The smiley gained huge popularity, became an international symbol of optimism
during the Vietnam War, and an icon in pop culture.

Creation of the simple smiley face led to tens of thousands of variations and
it has appeared on countless items ranging from clothing, home decor, stickers,
jewelry, and a vast collection of novelty items. Artist Dave Gibbons wrote: "It's
just a yellow field with three marks on it. It couldn't be more simple. And so to
that degree, it's empty. It's ready for meaning" (Stamp, 2013). This has made it an
invaluable tool for working with children in play therapy.

Rationale

A major goal of psychotherapy is to help children identify, express, and manage
emotions. Young children have cognitive and verbal limitations that make it difficult for them to do so. In addition, they often present with anxiety about talking

259

to the therapist. Feeling faces are an engaging, playful way to help children with these issues. They have a number of therapeutic benefits:

- *Communication.* Young children have a limited feelings vocabulary. Feeling faces provide a tangible tool for teaching them what feelings look and feel like, and for distinguishing among various feeling states. By pointing to pictures of feeling faces, the child is better able to express his/her emotions, which can lead to richer communication and enhanced functioning.

- *Emotional regulation.* The literature shows that individuals who use words to describe internal feeling states are more flexible and capable of regulating emotions in an adaptive way (Siegel, 2007). Feeling faces are an ideal way to teach children about feelings, which will help them express and regulate their internal experiences. Clearly, if a child does not have a name for something, it is more difficult for him/her to recognize it, understand it, and control it.

- *Relationship enhancement.* The ability to recognize feelings in others and express one's own feelings improves communication skills, cooperation, and compassion for others. These key elements contribute to positive peer relationships.

- *Diagnostic understanding.* Feeling faces help children discuss emotional experiences and situations. This provides the therapist with valuable information about the child's inner world and emotional needs.

Description

Ages

Children as young as 4 years can recognize the four basic emotions of glad, sad, mad, and afraid. By age 5 years they can identify the connection among emotional expressions, situations that cause specific emotions, and the consequences of such emotional expressions (Denham, 1986; Denham & Couchoud, 1990).

Materials

Posters or pictures of faces expressing various emotions (e.g., happy, sad, mad).

Techniques

Many therapists hang a feelings faces poster on the wall of the playroom for ready reference so that they can ask the child to point to a face most like how he/she is feeling or had felt in the past few days. Others start sessions by asking the child to draw a feeling face to show how he/she is feeling, or to describe a time when he/she had experienced that emotion. This will often lead to a discussion of antecedents and consequences of the feeling experience.

Variations

Flip-Flop Feeling Faces

This beanbag toss game by Discovery Toys is designed for children ages 4 years and up. It teaches children to understand facial expressions and enhances communication about emotions. Points are earned by landing a beanbag inside a bowl or by flipping a bowl. The game also encourages cooperative play, color/feeling associations such as an angry mad face, and social awareness.

Feelings Charades

In this group technique, feeling words are written on approximately 20 index cards (e.g., *cared*, *excited*, *brave*). Each child picks a card and silently acts out the feeling. The other members of the group have 1 minute to guess the feeling and share a time when they experienced it. Points may be earned for acting, guessing, or talking about the feeling. Feelings charades can also be played with a therapist, or at home with family members.

Feeling Stickers

Lowenstein (2001) introduced this technique for children of all ages. It requires a large piece of butcher-block paper and stickers with happy faces (happy feelings), sad faces (sad feelings), lizards (scared feelings), and stars (proud feelings). The therapist traces the child's body on the butcher-block paper and says, "We are going to use stickers to help us talk about feelings." The therapist then asks the child to talk about what makes him/her happy, sad, scared, and proud. After discussing each feeling the child is asked to place stickers on the outlined body to show where he/she feels those feelings in his/her body.

Feelings Ring Toss

Pam Dyson (n.d.) created this technique to help increase the feelings vocabulary of children ages 3 years and up. Materials needed include four plastic bottles (soda bottles are preferred), rice, sand or beans, clear packaging tape (wide enough to cover feeling faces), two each of four different feeling faces, four rings (made from 2 yards of clear tubing or four paper plates), glue gun, colored paper, markers or crayons, and scissors. Before the child's session, the therapist rinses and dries the bottles, pours rice or sand in the bottles to weight the bottoms so they won't tip, glues the lids back on, draws feeling faces (happy, sad, mad, and scared) onto colored paper, adds two feeling faces to each bottle, and covers them with clear packaging tape to secure. Paper plates with the center cut out could serve as rings. To play the game, the bottles are set in an open area. Standing several feet away, the child takes the four rings, one at a time, and tries to toss them around the bottles.

When the child gets a ring around a bottle, he/she calls out the name of the feeling face on that bottle. That feeling is then discussed.

Feelings Center

Benedict (1997) developed this technique as an adjunct to play therapy for preschool children presenting with disruptive classroom behaviors. The feelings center is set up in the classroom like other centers such as the reading corner or housekeeping corner. It is clearly demarcated from the other centers by dividers of low walls and/or decorations such as feelings posters. It is equipped with pillows or a beanbag chair; a mad pad where children can scribble vigorously; rubber stamps; a pounding toy; a collection of coloring sheets conveying feelings such as mad, sad, sacred, happy, and surprised; and other toys conducive to expression of emotions. The teacher or therapist acquaints children with the feelings center by reading a book about feelings to them and leading a discussion about ways to control upsetting feelings.

Empirical Findings

1. Using fMRI, Lieberman and colleagues (2007) showed a possible neuro-cognitive pathway by which labeling feelings helps to manage negative emotional experiences. Thirty participants looked at pictures of people with different emotional expressions. Below the picture of the face, they saw two feeling words, such as *angry* and *fearful*, and chose which emotion described the face, or they saw two names, such as "Harry" and "Sally," and chose the gender-appropriate name that matched the face. The researchers found that when the participants labeled the faces' emotions using words, a process they called "affect labeling," less activity occurred in the amygdala—an area associated with emotional distress. The participants also showed more activity in the right ventral lateral prefrontal cortex, the area associated with language and verbal expression. The authors concluded that verbalizing emotions activates the right ventral lateral prefrontal cortex that suppresses the areas of the brain connected with emotional pain. Lieberman noted, "In the same way you hit the brake when you're driving when you see a yellow light, when you put feelings into words, you seem to be hitting the brakes on your emotional responses" (UCLA College Report, 2010, p. 19).

2. Parker, Mathis, and Kupersmidt (2013) presented preschool children with an emotion recognition task that required them to identify emotions from facial expressions or body poses. The results showed that their accuracy in recognizing emotions on both photo tasks was related to teacher reports of their social skills.

3. Pennebaker, Kiecolt-Glaser, and Glaser (2008) showed that actively confronting upsetting experiences through talking or writing reduced negative effects of inhibition. In their experiment, 50 undergraduate college students were asked to write about either a traumatic experience or superficial topic for 4 consecutive days. Two measures of cellular immune-system function and health center visits suggested that confronting traumatic experiences was physically beneficial.

4. Philippot and Feldman (1990) found that preschoolers' ability to identify facial expressions of emotions correlated with their social competence.

Applications

Feeling faces can be used with various age groups and clinical populations. They are a tool for helping children recognize and express their emotional states, including anger, depression, fear, and anxiety. Feeling faces provide a way for therapists to help children discuss, release, and regulate their emotions instead of bottling them up or acting them out.

References

Benedict, H. E. (1997). The feelings center. In H. G. Kaduson & C. E. Schaefer (Eds.), *101 favorite play therapy techniques* (pp. 383–387). Northvale, NJ: Jason Aronson.

Denham, S. A. (1986). Social cognition, prosocial behavior, and emotion in preschoolers: Contextual variation. *Child Development, 56,* 197–201.

Denham, S. A., & Couchoud, E. (1990). Young preschoolers' ability to identify emotions in equivocal situations. *Child Study Journal, 20*(3), 153–165.

Dyson, P. (n.d.). Feelings ring toss. Retrieved from *http://stlplaytherapy.com/files/Feelings_Ring_Toss.pdf.*

Lieberman, M. D., Eisenberger, N. I., Crockett, M. J., Tom, S. M., Pfeifer, J. H., & Way, B. M. (2007). Putting feelings into words: Affect labeling disrupts amygdala activity in response to affective stimuli. *Psychological Science, 18*(5), 421–428.

Lowenstein, L. (2001). Feeling stickers. In H. G. Kaduson & C. E. Schaefer (Eds.), *101 more play therapy techniques* (pp. 88–91). Northvale, NJ: Jason Aronson.

Parker, A., Mathis, E. T., & Kupersmidt, J. B. (2013). How is this child feeling?: Preschool-aged children's ability to recognize emotion in faces and body poses. *Early Education and Development, 24,* 188–211.

Pennebaker, J. W., Kiecolt-Glaser, J. K., & Glaser, R. (2008). Disclosure of traumas and immune function: Health implications for psychotherapy. *Journal of Consulting and Clinical Psychology, 56*(2), 239–245.

Philippot, P., & Feldman, R. (1990). Age and social competence in preschoolers' decoding of facial expressions. *British Journal of Social Psychology, 29,* 43–54.

Siegel, D. (2007). *The mindful brain: Reflection and attunement in the cultivation of well-being.* New York: Norton.

Stamp, J. (2013). Who really invented the smiley face? *Smithsonian.* Retrieved from *www.smithsonianmag.com/arts-culture/who-really-invented-the-smiley-face-2058483/?no-ist.*

What happens when we put feelings into words? (2010, Winter). *UCLA College Report, 13,* 18–19. Retrieved from *www.college.ucla.edu/report/uclacollegereport13.pdf.*

57

Suitcase Playroom

"What a funny bag!" Michael said. There was nothing inside. But
the next moment Mary Poppins took out a white apron, a large cake
of soap, a tooth-brush, a packet of hairpins, a bottle of perfume and
a small armchair. Jane and Michael were shocked.
—P. L. Travers

Introduction

Child therapists often sublet or share office space, work in hospitals, schools, or
homes, or travel between offices. Consequently, they frequently do not have a place
to store and organize play materials. Cassell (1979) introduced the suitcase playroom for child therapists who lack a permanent playroom. She recommended a
prescribed list of toys and art materials known to promote self-expression and aid
in the therapeutic process. Three suitcases are filled with these materials, making
play therapy more portable and readily available to children.

Rationale

The suitcase playroom enables child therapists to meet the needs of children who
may not otherwise receive services due to lack of a playroom or office space. The
suitcase play materials as prescribed by Cassell (1979), includes toys and art materials for self-expression, role play, creative thinking, fantasy, metaphorical teaching, mastery, and relationship enhancement. In addition, the suitcase playroom
provides a number of specific therapeutic benefits:

• *Positive emotion.* Young children are thrilled by the idea of a suitcase containing toys and play materials. Exploring the contents is an engaging activity that
captures their interest and cooperation.

- *Working alliance.* The fact that the therapist brings toys to the session gives the child a sense that he/she is cared for and valued. It shows the child that the therapist plans for the sessions and is committed to the child's treatment. These factors contribute to a working alliance.

- *Communication.* By selecting toys based on the child's interests, developmental needs, and abilities, the therapist communicates understanding, empathy, and compassion. These toys in turn, enable the child to communicate and work through feelings, thoughts, and needs.

- *Problem solving/creative thinking.* Seeing that the therapist carries supplies to the sessions shows the child that challenges can be overcome with creativity, planning, and effort. The reward of playing with the toys conveys that facing challenges can bring about pleasure and great rewards.

Description

Ages: Four and up

Materials

Materials needed for Cassell's (1979) suitcase playroom include one large suitcase (20½ × 7 inches), two small suitcases in different colors (5½ × 10 inches), portable stage, portable furnished dollhouse with handle (about 9 × 15 inches when closed).

The large suitcase holds:

- One small box filled with 15 miniature cars and trucks (including emergency, construction, and mail vehicles) and a set of small miniature dolls to fit the dollhouse.
- One large box filled with Lego blocks, and 6-inch wooden figures comprising two families (African American and Caucasian) and community workers.
- One large box filled with army toys including soldiers, four tanks, four trucks, two jeeps, and assorted small field guns, and a dollhouse bathroom with tub, toilet, and washbowl.
- Art materials including a large pad, crayons, markers, plasticene, and clay (which are placed in the zippered flap of the suitcase).

The two small suitcases hold:

- One doll family each (Caucasian and African American).
- Family puppets with plastic heads (including a baby with removable bottle).
- Other plastic-headed puppets including a doctor, a worker, and a police officer.
- A variety of animal puppets that foster identification and self-expression. These would include a fierce crocodile, a cuddly skunk, and a furry brown bear.

Before displaying the suitcase material, it is important that the therapist physically define the play space by laying down a rug or other object for the child to play on.

Variations

Play Cabinet

Kuntz (2003) introduced this technique for children from infancy to adolescence who undergo long-term hospitalizations. The use of a play cabinet in the children's unit provides hospitalized children with therapeutic play experiences that are integrated into their daily schedule. The cabinet is filled with blankets, pillows, and age-appropriate toys, books, and music that can turn a hospital room into a therapeutic space. Including play into daily care can help medical personnel understand the child's development and emotions, and can help children communicate and play out fears and anxieties. Kuntz notes that a supply of toys for four age groups can be stored in the cabinet: infants, toddlers and preschoolers, school-age children, and adolescents. Toys for infants include mats, balls, toys, puppets, mobiles, and rattles. Toys for toddlers and preschool children include blocks, cars, carts, dress-up clothes, cups, dishes, dolls and sets, push-and-pull toys, puzzles, rocking horses, tool benches and water-play items, and stamps and ink. Toys for school-age children include action figures, board games, puzzles, soft balls, and craft kits. Adolescent materials include games, videos, crafts, mosaics, journals, jewelry kits, stamps, inks, and video games. Materials for all age groups include soft blankets and pillowcases; age-appropriate books and music; and a wide variety of art materials such as crayons, markers, and paints.

Deluxe Rolling Play Therapy Kit/Mobile Play Therapy Kit with Rolling Duffle

This set available from childtherapytoys.com is for the traveling therapist, or the therapist with multiple offices. It includes a portable rolling duffle equipped with a tarp, dollhouse, dollhouse family (with a choice of skin tone), male or female doll, card game sets (Old Maid, Animal Rummy, and Go Fish), Checkers set, foam balls, the Social and Emotional Competence Game, military accessories, tool set, modeling clay, wood blocks, a dish/cookware set, food set, Silly Putty, play money, doctor kit, cellphone, markers, doodle pads, set of soldiers, dinosaurs, domestic cat and domestic dog, wild west set, and a small "How are you feeling?" poster.

Empirical Findings

This technique is in need of empirical research.

Applications

The suitcase playroom can be adapted to work with children and adolescents of all ages with a wide variety of presenting problems. Because the suitcase can be filled with whatever toys or materials are needed, the benefits of this technique are endless. The suitcase playroom enables the child therapist to meet the needs of children in underserved communities, in disaster-struck environments, and settings where toys may not be available. It also enables educators and experienced clinicians to provide hands-on training for aspiring play therapists.

References

Cassell, S. (1979). The suitcase playroom. In C. E. Schaefer (Ed.), *Therapeutic use of child's play* (pp. 413–414). Northvale, NJ: Jason Aronson.

Kuntz, N. (2003). Play cabinet. In H. G. Kaduson & C. E. Schaefer (Eds.), *101 favorite play therapy techniques* (Vol. 3, pp. 263–267). Lanham, MD: Jason Aronson.

58

Play Therapy Rituals

By such ritual acts we announce who we are, and, in the sharing and
re-enactment, bind our attachment to one another.
—KEVIN CHANDLER

Introduction

A ritual is a ceremony, procedure, or action performed in a routine way. Rituals
are seen in the way religious services, marital unions, and funerals are conducted;
the way holidays and milestones are celebrated; and the way families share meals
and end the day. The therapeutic value of rituals in psychotherapy is often over-
looked in favor of the content of the sessions. Rituals in play therapy provide
children with predictability and a sense of safety and containment. This serves to
reduce anxiety and foster a sense of personal control (Gallo-Lopez, 2006). Many
children in play therapy are impulsive and find transitions between activities difficult to manage. They need assistance settling down as the sessions commence
and disengaging from a play activity when a session is over. Rituals in play therapy
commonly include beginning therapy, starting and ending sessions, celebrating client progress, and terminating therapy.

Rationale

Rituals serve many purposes and have a variety of benefits when used in play
therapy, including:

• *Therapeutic alliance.* Rituals for beginning play therapy serve to reduce
resistance; establish a therapeutic alliance; and help children feel comfortable,
respected, and secure. They show children that the therapist is consistent, reliable,
and trustworthy; make therapy familiar; and help children feel safe and cared for.

• *Belonging/group cohesiveness.* Rituals such as snack time, playing the child's favorite or made-up game, and circle time in group counseling promote a sense of belonging and group cohesiveness.

• *Positive emotion.* Rituals such as parties or snacks are enjoyable and contribute to the child's sense of well-being. They can also serve as a break from reality for overburdened children. In addition, providing food serves as a source of nurturance that can be very healing for children with histories of loss and impoverishment.

• *Transition issues.* Rituals for beginning sessions help children transition from their everyday lives to the therapy room. They signal "Now we begin" and help children settle into the session and refocus on the task of therapy. Likewise, rituals for ending sessions prepare children for leaving and provide closure. They give children an opportunity to process feelings about the session and help them leave feeling calm, relaxed, and positive.

• *Safety.* Being able to predict what is coming next helps children feel competent. Knowing how and when situations are taking place helps children feel prepared and grounded. This is especially helpful for children with unstable homes who commonly experience insecurity and a sense of floundering.

• *Self-esteem.* Rituals for celebrating when children meet treatment goals or other life milestones are enjoyable and give children a sense of pride. This empowers them to meet future goals and fosters feelings of competence and self-esteem.

• *Termination issues.* The ending phase of treatment is an opportunity to help children process their accomplishments, their past separations and losses, and their future. Termination rituals help to make the ending of treatment tangible, highlight the child's accomplishments, instill pride, provide a healthy model for saying goodbye, address loss issues, and anticipate how to solve problems in the future (Cangelosi, 1997). Thus, it is essential to have a termination ritual and to give the child 2–4 weeks to process the end of therapy sessions.

Description

Ages

All ages

Techniques

Rituals are conducted in various ways depending on their purpose. A basic ritual for beginning therapy or starting sessions on a positive note is to greet the child warmly with a smile, eye contact, and saying the child's name. The greeting ritual typically includes an attempt to initiate a verbal interaction by asking a question or making a comment ("I like your smile!"). The therapist might also offer some fruit juice boxes and little snacks because some children come right from school and are so hungry that it is difficult for them to focus during the session. Other rituals to begin a session might include removing shoes, exploring toys, introducing a drawing activity, exchanging a "high five," or playing a familiar game. The squiggle game and other projective techniques are a great way to start sessions because they are enjoyable, interactive, and provide the therapist with information about the child's thoughts and inner world. The therapist might also play ball; tell a story; or offer a blanket, pillow, or stuffed animals to comfort the child. In groups, helpful rituals for beginning treatment include taking a place in the circle, playing a trust game, or discussing why the children came to the group.

Rituals for celebrating the child's accomplishment in play therapy include having a party or giving the child a certificate or present. Rituals for ending sessions might entail having a snack; bibliotherapy; doing a simple drawing activity to wind down; and selecting a small prize from a treasure chest, such as a balloon, party favor, or sticker. Termination rituals might take the form of a farewell party designed by both therapist and child; a review of the child's accomplishments in therapy; a discussion of mutual feelings around saying goodbye; and a certificate of achievement or gift, such as a transitional object, from the therapist. Another possibility is a ritual box for the child to take home, filled with products from intervention work done in the playroom since the first session.

Variations

Creative Cleanup Technique

Pehrsson (2003) introduced this technique to address the issue of cleanup at the end of play therapy sessions. Five to 10 minutes before the end of the session, the therapist tells the child, "Our time is almost up for today. We have just a little more time left. And now I am for cleaning and you are for finishing." The therapist then proceeds to clean up the room and allows time for the child to complete the activity. If a limit is needed, the therapist says, "There are no more new toys for using during cleanup." When the room is clean the therapist tells the child that time is up for the day and asks if the child would like to open the door.

The Little Leaf Transition Ritual

Cerio (2001) developed this ritual to help children transition from the play therapy session back to the classroom or home. It is especially useful for children who become overstimulated or have difficulty discontinuing with play. The therapist tells the child a metaphorical/relaxation story entitled *The Little Leaf* in a sing-song type of intonation, alternating the pitch from high to medium to low, and the volume from moderate to whispers. This together with the content of the story about a leaf that falls to the ground and attains a state of calm—induces a state of relaxation in the child. The child is then told, "Now when you return to class, you will continue to feel relaxed and alert" (p. 40).

The Title of Therapy

This technique (Dee, 2001) helps children recognize and verbalize their experiences in therapy and to process the effects it had on them. In the final two counseling sessions, the therapist presents the child with all of the drawings he/she completed throughout treatment. The child is encouraged to discuss the events that were occurring and how he/she was feeling at the time of each drawing in addition to current feelings about the drawings. The therapist then asks the child to title each drawing and places them in chronological order on the floor. The child discusses similarities and differences in the drawings and other relevant issues. He/she then decides whether to take the artwork home or leave it with the therapist.

Saying Goodbye—Breaking the Links in a Chain

Lawrence (2003) developed this technique to help children ages 4–8 years prepare for the ending of therapy. Three or 4 weeks before the child's last therapy session, the child makes a chain using strips of colored paper. The child or therapist then writes the date on the first link, and the dates of upcoming sessions on the other links. Each time the child arrives for a session, he/she breaks away the link for that session, making note of how many sessions are remaining.

Hand Drawings

In this technique, the therapist and child outline their hands next to each other on a sheet of paper. This souvenir provides the child with a reminder of the therapeutic partnership and a source of ego support after treatment ends (Shelby, 1996). The therapist makes a copy of the sheet to let the child know that he/she will be remembered.

Goodbye Gifts

The therapist may want to give the child a present when completing treatment. When choosing a present it is important to consider the message it conveys and the ways in which it may influence the child—for example, giving a journal or sketch pad promotes the importance of self-expression and encourages the child to continue exploring and expressing feelings, thoughts, ideas, and images. Gifts of this nature also show children that the therapist values their feelings and thoughts. Similarly, giving the child who is an avid reader a book by his/her favorite author conveys that the therapist heard the child's preferences and promotes his/her interests. The therapist may also choose to give a gift directly from the playroom that the child enjoyed playing with or that had significant meaning during the treatment—for example, this therapist (DC) gave an adolescent her favorite magic wand from the playroom when she left treatment to go away to college. The wand helped the girl discuss problems when she started treatment and she often played with it or made wishes with it as an adolescent. The wand was given to the girl as a reminder of our work together, a source of comfort during her transition to college, and as a metaphor for her to continue expressing her wishes and needs.

Empirical Findings

1. Eilam, Izhar, and Mort (2011) found that basketball players, animals in captivity, and patients with OCD use ritualistic behaviors to manage stress and anxiety associated with situations in which control is lacking. In a healthy use of rituals, the researchers noted that basketball players completing a free throw frequently engaged in a ritual of bouncing the ball a precise number of times before throwing it. According to the researchers, this improved the players' focus, concentration and control of their actions.

2. Norton and Gino (2014) found that engaging in rituals lessens grief caused by both life-changing losses (death of a loved one or a breakup) and more mundane ones (losing a lottery). In one experiment, participants were asked to write about the death of a loved one or the end of a close relationship. Participants in a second group also wrote about a ritual they performed after experiencing the loss. The researchers found that people who wrote about engaging in a ritual reported feeling less grief than did those who only wrote about the loss.

The researchers also examined the power of rituals for reducing disappointment about losing the lottery. Participants were told that they were part of a random drawing in which they could win $200 and were asked to write about the ways they would use the money. After the random draw, the winner left and the remaining participants were divided into two groups. One group engaged in a four-step ritual while the control group engaged in a generic drawing activity. Participants who performed a ritual after losing the lottery reported feeling less grief.

Applications

Rituals help children in treatment cope better with the stress of transitions and change. Beginning rituals provide structure and predictability that helps insecure, shy, and slow-to-warm-up children adjust to starting treatment. Using rituals in a consistent way throughout treatment gives children with ADHD or unstable, tumultuous, or abusive backgrounds a sense of calm, predictability, and security, and fosters healthy attachments. Celebratory rituals provide a relief from stressful feelings for children with loss and trauma issues and promote self-esteem and pride for children who attain treatment goals. Closing rituals for ending a session are particularly important for children with attachment disorders and separation anxiety. Finally, termination rituals instill a sense of accomplishment, pride, and hope, and give all children in treatment time to process their feelings about ending the therapeutic relationship.

References

Cangelosi, D. (1997). *Saying goodbye in child psychotherapy: Planned, unplanned and premature endings*. Northvale, NJ: Jason Aronson.

Cerio, J. (2001). The little leaf transition ritual. In H. G. Kaduson & C. E. Schaefer (Eds.), *101 more play therapy techniques* (pp. 37–40). Northvale, NJ: Jason Aronson.

Dee, R. (2001). The title of therapy. In H. G. Kaduson & C. E. Schaefer (Eds.), *101 more play therapy techniques* (pp. 146–149). Northvale, NJ: Jason Aronson.

Eilam, D., Izhar, R., & Mort, J. (2011). Threat detection: Behavioral practices in animals and humans. *Neuroscience and Biobehavioral Reviews*, *35*(4), 999–1006.

Gallo-Lopez, L. (2006). A creative play therapy approach to the group treatment of young sexually abused children. In H. G. Kaduson & C. E. Schaefer (Eds.), *Short-term play therapy for children* (pp. 245–272). New York: Guilford Press.

Lawrence, B. (2003). Saying goodbye: Breaking the links on a chain. In H. G. Kaduson & C. E. Schaefer (Eds.), *101 favorite play therapy techniques* (Vol. 3, pp. 413–416). Lanham, MD: Jason Aronson.

Norton, M., & Gino, F. (2014). Rituals alleviate grieving for loved ones, lovers and lotteries. *Journal of Experimental Psychology General*, *143*(1), 266–272.

Pehrsson, D. E. (2003). The creative clean-up technique. In H. G. Kaduson & C. E. Schaefer (Eds.), *101 favorite play therapy techniques* (Vol. 3, pp. 413–416). Lanham, MD: Jason Aronson.

Shelby, J. (1996, July). *Post-traumatic play therapy for survivors of acute abuse and community violence*. Paper presented at the 11th annual Summer Play Therapy Seminar, Hackensack, NJ.

Index